What Yo Doctor Isn't Telling You About Back Pain

RAJ BANERJEE, D.C.

Requests for permission to use any part of this book should be addressed to:
Permission • 7486 Crystal Lake Drive • Cordova, TN 38018

To order the book go to http://www.DrBanerjee

Printed in United States of America

First printing 2007

ISBN 13: 978-0-9801629-0-5

BANERJEE, RAJ
What Your Doctor Isn't Telling You About Back Pain
by Raj Banerjee, D.C.

Editing by Marcia Gervase, redline8express@yahoo.com

Cover & interior design / layout by Michele Bryant
www.michelesdesign.com • 407-381-1288 • michele@michelesdesign.com

What Your Doctor Isn't Telling You About Back Pain

The 'Breakthrough' Whole Mind-Body Approach to Natural Back Pain Relief

RAJ BANERJEE, D.C.

ACKNOWLEDGEMENTS

My first appreciation is to my parents, who have unfailingly supported and encouraged me. For their unconditional love that has made all this possible. My father, Dr. Shyamal Banerjee, a scientist and a scholar, is a great teacher and a role model to me.

My mother, Attreyi Banerjee, continues to be my best cheerleader, is the best and most amazing mother a son can hope to have, makes it all worth it.

Special thanks to my friend, and my mentor Todd Taylor, who gave me great advice, encouragement, and motivation and helped me make this a better book.

My patients, who have taught me more than I can ever hope to teach them.

And finally, God and my Guru Sri Ramakrishna, for the guidance and infinite blessing I have been given and for using me as an instrument for healing.

TABLE OF CONTENTS

CHAPTER 9   Passive Therapies for Back Pain . . . 101

CHAPTER 10 Invasive Conservative Treatments for Back Pain 129

CHAPTER 11   Alternative Treatments 147

CHAPTER 12   Chiropractic Care Can Stop Pain and Help Restore Good Health. . . . 165

For other books and programs by
Dr. Raj Banerjee, including

*"Dr. Banerjee's Guide to Hormone Imbalance:
Discover Simple Steps to Rebuild Your Life."*

FREE Video Newsletter, please visit:

http://www.DrBanerjee.com

You will also discover secrets:

- How to Reverse Chronic Fatigue

- How to Stop Depression Dead In
  It's Tracks

- How to Destroy Pain & Live Happy
  Without Pills

- How to Stop Dieting and Lose Weight
  Automatically

- Medical Secrets Doctors Never Mention

- *And Much, Much, More ...*

Please visit:
http://www.DrBanerjee.com

Understanding Back Pain

Since you are reading this book, you or a loved one may be suffering from the horrible condition called *low back pain* that strikes millions of Americans each year.

What I will reveal inside this book may show you how to finally rid yourself of low back pain without drugs or surgery, so please be sure to read everything here—it may be the most important information on back pain that you've read in a long time!

Before we get started, think if you have ever asked yourself any or all of these questions:

- ❖ Why does my back hurt?
- ❖ Why doesn't the pain just go away?
- ❖ Why can't I just be like normal people?
- ❖ How bad can this physical condition get?
- ❖ Will I eventually be crippled?
- ❖ Will I ever be able to live the life I used to?

If any one of these problems or concerns is creating a situation that affects the quality of your life, then you need to go through this book and really understand back pain and how to beat it.

Nothing Is Worse Than Feeling Great Mentally— Wanting to Take in All Life Has to Offer—Only to Have Your Natural Enthusiasm and Drive Squashed Because Your Back Hurts and The Pain Just Won't Go Away!

Isn't it sad to feel so alive and full of vigor, and not be able to do all the things you want to do because the low back pain you suffer from is so pervasive, so intrusive, and so unfair?

Don't you feel downright angry because this pain, these symptoms, just won't go away?

If you do, it's only normal. After all, who wants to be burdened with carrying a load of discomfort, and living life through an all-encompassing fog of pain. Pain that's always there when you stand up, sit down, lie down, or even bend over. Pain that always rears its head, no matter how hard you try to ignore it.

It's natural for people to try to tough it out and get on with their lives. "If I ignore it long enough, it will go away ..." Unfortunately, this isn't the case. Ignoring your pain will only make it worse over time. What was only a mild pain a year or month ago, may become a chronic, crippling pain years down the road.

You see, low back pain is so bad because it sort of sneaks up on you. The real cause of the pain you're feeling right now may have happened years ago. It may have been such a small injury you might not have noticed it. Or maybe you felt a slight pain, but it went away after a day or week so you didn't think much of it.

And slowly, over the years, as you continued to do your normal activities, that old injury has gotten worse and worse without you being aware of it. After a time, the straws slowly built up until one day they broke the camel's back. Maybe what finally put you over the edge was that heavy chair you tried to lift, or that time you bent over too quickly, or any one of a hundred things.

Whatever it was,

The Fact Is You Are Suffering from Low Back Pain and You Don't Have to Suffer Anymore!

So what do you do? What choices do you have? We know you may have already tried getting some relief from over-the-counter drugs, or maybe you met with your private doctor. But do you know what is causing your back pain?

There are many reasons why you have back pain. This book will guide you through what to do and what not to do to fix your back pain. I know how terrible it is to have back pain. The scary thing is that most of the time back pain can creep up on you without you noticing it. Then all of a sudden it hits you one day. Maybe it was something you tried to lift, or maybe it was something you reached for. And suddenly the muscles tighten and your back stiffens. Many patients tell me that their back pain started many years ago and now it is a chronic pain that never goes away.

Back pain can be scary, just like any other pain. Many of my patients will have movement anxiety. This is where they limit themselves and limit their movements because they're afraid their back will give out on them. It is also scary when you go to a doctor and you don't know what to expect. He may start ordering different test. Or maybe describe things that you don't understand. After you've gone through this book, you'll know exactly what to expect and you'll know what to ask the doctor. This book will empower you so that you can be your own health advocate.

How I Help People with Back Pain

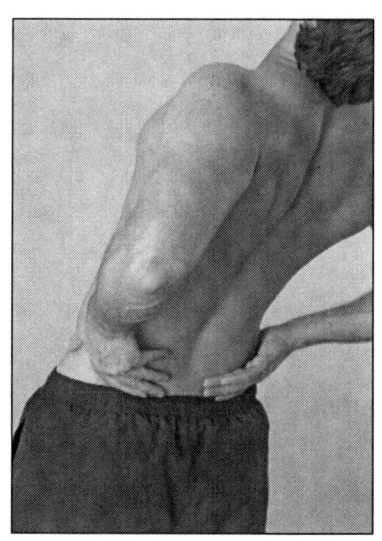

I treat back pain differently than other doctors. I use a whole mind-body hormone approach. I also use a multidisciplinary approach. So when someone comes in for back pain, not only will I talk to them about their back pain, but I will also talk to them about their lifestyle and the kind of stress they are experiencing, including how they handle stress. I'll talk to them about their diet and nutrition. I may even test them to see how balanced their hormones are. So I treat the whole person, not just the back, because that is the only way to get the best results.

With the multidisciplinary approach, you are in an environment where there is a medical doctor, a massage therapist, a physical therapist, a chiropractor, all working together to help you. With this approach, I've been able to help many patients avoid surgery to correct back pain.

When you go through this book, you will notice that this book is not just about back pain, but how to live a life full of vibrant health. You'll notice that I go through many emotional and physical causes of back pain. You will also understand the best ways to fix back pain. I'll talk about common causes, common treatments, and help you put together a plan that you can follow.

This book is designed to be easy to follow. To get the most out of this book, I recommend you read the parts that interest you most and also follow along with the lessons from my Inner Circle Group. You will see a huge improvement in your health if you do that. You may want to read the book a few times to let everything really sink in. I have taken a lot of my personal tips and strategies that I use with my own patients and made them available to you.

It's not necessary that you read the book from cover to cover. What is necessary is that you subscribe to my free video newsletter at www.drbanerjee.com That way I can keep you updated on new breakthroughs and techniques to transform your health.

Why Low Back Pain Confuses Doctors and Chiropractors …

Back pain is a huge problem. It affects almost everyone, doctors included. Most doctors just don't seem to have the right answer for this problem. If you're reading this book, it's a fair guess that you or someone close to you suffer from back pain. You're looking for answers to resolve this problem. If you have been looking for answers for awhile, you can see how frustrating it can be to find the right treatments or the right exercises that will solve your back pain problem once and for all.

It is hugely frustrating that every back pain sufferer seems to have his own opinion about back pain. Some may swear by chiropractors, while others go to physical therapists, and others opt for surgery.

Why is there so much confusion about back pain? Why does one doctor say one thing and another doctor say something else? Why is it that even though this is such a common condition, healthcare professionals cannot come together with one sure answer? If you've spent any time researching the topic of back pain, you will begin to understand how confusing it can be.

I believe there are three reasons why there is so much confusion about effective treatments for back pain. The number one reason is that most of time the true cause of the back pain is not known. And the reason why doctors disagree on treatments is because their diagnoses are different. The third and most important reason why back pain treatments may not be effective is because the doctor is not taking care of the whole body. She may take X-rays or MRIs of your spine, but she really needs to be looking at you as a person. The whole, dynamic you.

It's as if a doctor has a little picture of what is going on, and he assumes what works for one person will work for you. But that is not how the body works. Everyone is not the same. Everyone is individual, and so the same treatment that works for one person may not work for you.

I'm going to start building different foundations for you. We will touch on many different topics that contribute to your health. Not only are you going to learn how to fix your back pain, you will learn how to be a healthy, energetic, and a more balanced person. And that will decrease inflammation and make your body stronger.

And that will decrease inflammation and make your body stronger.

What Is Back Pain?

What actually is back pain? Is it just pain in your back or something more? Pain can include many different symptoms and can express itself in many different ways.

As we discussed earlier, back pain has many causes. These causes can be anything physical, emotional, or even a hormonal imbalance. If you don't look at the whole person, you're likely to miss what is actually causing the back pain. I will discuss these components in greater detail in later chapters. But unfortunately it is a fact that most healthcare professionals will ignore either the emotional or the hormonal aspect of this condition.

It is also safe to assume that in the majority of the cases of back pain, most healthcare professionals will not investigate what is actually causing the pain. And in many instances, the pain will go away regardless of the treatment, because our bodies are so dynamic and so adaptable.

Two of the most common causes for back pain are misaligned vertebra and muscle imbalances. These are example of the physical aspects of low back pain. In this book you will discover some easy ways to correct your muscle imbalances. Muscle imbalances can affect the muscles and ligaments and tendons in your body. If supporting structures in your back become weak, your discs can be affected.

The whole thing about back pain is that it is a process. You'll beat your back pain once you know where you are in that process and find workable solutions to stop and reverse the process.

When the discs in your spine are affected, you can get disk herniation and disc protrusions. The disc acts as a cushion that lies between each vertebra of your spine. These disk problems can also result in pinched nerves. The pain produced by disc herniation and protrusions are diverse. Sometime the pain will go down your leg; sometimes the pain can be burning. Other times the pain can have numbness associated with it. It can also be something completely different.

Another reason people have back pain that most doctors miss is chronic stress and how stress affects your hormones. Sometimes emotional trauma can actually initiate a back pain. Other times, back pain may start due to physical reasons, and emotional stresses will prolong or worsen that pain. Knowing how to handle stress, and also seeing how your hormones are affecting your body, are crucial to healing back pain.

The Practical Way to Cure Back Pain

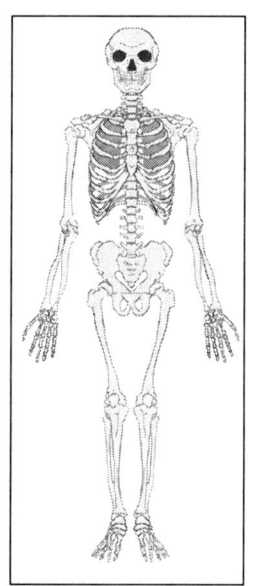

Do not be discouraged. Know that you're not alone in your attempts to understand the mechanisms of back pain. Your back pain will get better, if you give it a chance. Become your own health advocate. Learn as much as you can. Find the information that really clicks with you and make it practical.

Try the stretches that appeal to you. Do the strengthening exercises that work for your body type. Try out the dietary changes that I recommend in the Inner Circle Group. Everyone has to start somewhere.

When you get into a pattern of healthy habits, other things will become much easier. You will understand the true mechanism of pain in the mechanism of healing. It will be easier to find a treatment and a health practitioner who can work with you. You'll never have to be dependent on anyone else.

Can Your Back Pain Get Better?

It is true that back pain is very common and most of the time your body has the ability to take care of it. The ability to finally resolve back pain is actually very good. And once you learn some simple and easy strategies to make yourself healthy, you'll start to see the light at the end of the tunnel.

There is also the chance that your back pain won't get better on its own. Chances are if you're reading this book your back pain has not gotten better. You may have experienced flare-ups that come and go and you may have no idea why. Maybe you may have a chronic kind of pain, where it's nagging and irritating over a long period of time. Or you may have some intense sharp pain that makes you freeze in your tracks.

Perhaps you have muscle spasms so intense that it's hard for you to even walk or move around. Or maybe you have had back pain surgeries that failed to relieve your symptoms.

Back pain can be very frustrating for you and your loved ones. Finding out what the real underlining cause is even more important. If you don't find out what's actually causing your pain, then whatever treatment you do is only guesswork. It might work, it might not. The first step to fix your back pain is to discover its cause.

After you discover what's causing it, the best treatment is to treat the whole body. Not just your back pain. You want to take a holistic approach to your problem and see the big picture.

Any kind of surgery should always be the last resort. After you've exhausted every other treatment option, then you can think about opting for spinal surgery. In my experience spinal surgery is very ineffective. If the problem is caught early and the correct treatment is given, then most of the time the back pain will resolve. Even in very chronic cases. Now if there are severe trauma, fractures, and other such injuries, surgery is called for. But in a majority of back pain cases, surgery can be prevented.

A Few Things You Should Know About Your Spine

In this chapter, we will help you get familiar with your spine's anatomy so you will be able to ask better questions, which will get you better answers, and therefore the treatment you really need.

A few things you should know about your spine:

1. **Hundreds of muscles and ligaments support your spine.** Then all of these muscles and ligaments work as they should, it creates a very strong structure. Also your spine is very flexible, able to twist and bend while supporting your head and torso.

2. **Most of the back pain cases that doctors see can be corrected by creating balance in your body.** If your doctor rules out a tumor, pain that is due to anything life-threatening, or something that requires immediate surgery, then creating muscle balance, mind-body balance, and hormone balance will get rid of your back pain.

3. **Surgery should be the absolute last option.** You need to learn about and try every option before agreeing to surgery because surgery is rarely necessary to get rid of pain. And once you do surgery there is no going back and undoing it. Your body will never be the same.

4. **Simply find the true cause for your pain and fix it.** If you have multiple sources of imbalances, start with the major ones and slowly create balance in the different systems in your body.

Why Your Spine Is So Important

Have you ever wondered what the function and purpose of your spine is? Your spine:

1. **Creates support for your body.**   Muscles and ligaments attach to it. Your spine holds your head up, and it holds your torso up. It creates stability and allows you to do simple things to very complex activities such as dance. It serves as a foundation for your body.

2. **Creates flexibility.**   Can you imagine if your spine were like a straight, rigid rod? You would have no movement at all. Your spine is very flexible, allowing you to bend backward, forward, side-to-side, twist, and combinations of these movements.

3. **Protects your delicate spinal cord and nerves.**   Your spinal cord and nerves serve as a highway that relays messages from your brain to your end organs like your muscles, organs, or other tissues. Your spine protects these very delicate nerve structures while you move and bend. Did you know that the amount of pressure exerted from a dime is enough to block 90% of nerve signal? That's how delicate we are talking about.

4. **Has a specific structure for a specific function.**   If there is imbalance in the structure then the function will suffer. For example, think about a regular chair. The structure is that it has four legs. The function for the legs is to hold the person sitting up. If you were to do something to one of the legs, the function would suffer.

Spine 101: Anatomy of Your Spine

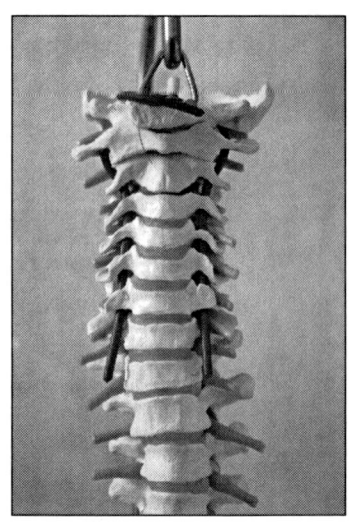

The rest of the chapter we will discuss the anatomy of the spine. Your spine can be divided into the following structures:

- ❖ the spinal column
- ❖ the vertebrae
- ❖ the discs
- ❖ the facet joints
- ❖ the ligaments
- ❖ the spinal canal

* the sacrum and coccyx

* the sacroiliac joint

* the nerves

* the muscles

The spinal column

When you look at your spine from front to back, it should look straight. Your skull sits on top of the cervical vertebrae, your hips align with your lumbar spine, and there are no curvatures. When you look at your spine from the side, you should have three flowing curves that look like an S-shape. The first curve is a cervical curve, then the thoracic curve, and finally the lumbar curve.

You have 24 bones in your spine stacked on top of each other. They are called vertebrae (plural) or vertebra (singular).

* Your neck or your cervical part of your spine contains seven bones. These bones support and stabilize your head and protect the delicate nerves that run from your brain to the rest of your body. These vertebrae are named C1, C2, C3, C4, C5, C6, and C7. C1 is at the top just under your head.

* The thoracic part which makes up the upper- and mid-back contains 12 bones. These vertebrae are referred to as T1 to T12.

* The lumbar portion has 5 bones and it makes up your lower back. They are referred to as L1 to L5. Some of the strongest muscles and ligaments reside here. The lumbar curve supports the rest of your body and majority of the weight.

When you have good posture and muscle balance in your spine, your ear, shoulder, and hip align to make a straight line. Having good posture means to have these curves in their proper place.

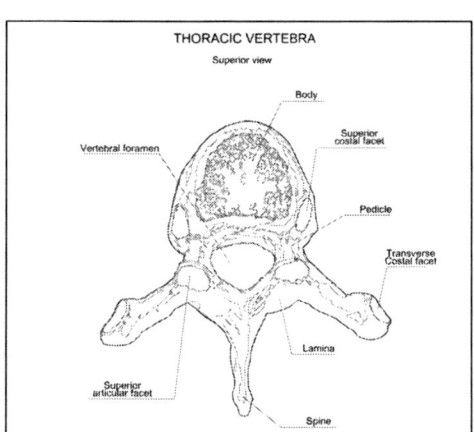

THORACIC VERTEBRA
Superior view

Body

Superior costal facet

Vertebral foramen

Pedicle

Transverse Costal facet

Lamina

Superior articular facet

Spine

Vertebrae: The Bones of Your Back

There are three parts to the vertebrae: the vertebral body, the transverse process, and the spinous process. Your spine consists of 24 of these vertebrae.

The vertebral body is the largest part of the vertebra. It is in the front end and is cushioned by the discs. The bony bumps that you can feel on your back are the spinous process. This is where many of the spinal muscles that control your spine's movement attach. Also in the diagram notice the spinal canal. This is where your spinal cord passes through.

The Discs

You will find a disc between each of the vertebral bodies. The disc acts as your spine's shock absorbers. The way the discs are designed allows the bony vertebra to move back and forth, giving your spine incredible flexibility.

There are two parts that make up the disc.

1. **Nucleus propulsus**   This is the center of your disc. It is made up of mostly water, making it very flexible and spongy. This spongy center creates flexibility in between each vertebra and provides a shock-absorbing cushion to the structures of your spine.

2. **Annulus fibrosis**   This is the tough outer layer of the disc that actually attaches to the vertebra, actually holding them together. The annulus fiber is a very strong and tough material and has a crisscross design to give it more strength.

The Facet Joints

The facet joints, known also as the gliding joints in your vertebrae, are considered synovium joints because between the joints are joint capsules that consist of a smooth lining called synovium. The job of the synovium is to create synovial fluid in the joint capsule. The synovial fluid lubricates the joint so it can have smooth movement.

The Ligaments

Ligaments are strong bands of fibrous tissue that attach one bone to another bone. Ligaments also contain pain fibers. Two of the major ligaments in your spine are 1. The anterior longitudinal ligament, and 2. The posterior longitudinal ligament.

These two ligaments go up and down your whole spine and attach the vertebrae together. Ligaments help with motion of your spine while providing flexibility.

The Spinal Canal

The delicate spinal cord passes through this opening. The opening is made because the vertebrae are aligned on top of each other.

The Sacrum and Coccyx

Below the lumbar vertebrae, there are five more vertebrae that are fused together. This forms the back of your pelvis and the lowest part of your lumbosacral curve. These five vertebrae make up the sacrum.

Most people have five lumbar vertebrae and five fused sacral vertebrae. But in some people they may have six lumbar vertebra and four fused sacral vertebrae. Even if you have six lumbar vertebrae, it is very unlikely that your back pain is due to just this.

The coccyx is the very bottom part of your spine. It is attached to the very bottom of the sacrum and consists of three to five small bones. The layman's term for this structure is the tailbone.

The Sacroiliac Joints

The joints that attach the sacrum to the iliac bones are called the sacroiliac joints.

The Nerves

The spinal cord is made up of nerves that extend from the brain, pass through the spinal canal, and then out to various parts of the body. The spinal cord is surrounded by the cerebral spinal fluid (CSF). This is the same fluid that surrounds the brain. Cerebral spinal fluid helps protect the spinal cord inside the spinal canal.

The nerve roots are the parts where the nerves exit the spine and go to their target end organ. These nerves go to everywhere in your body. They send the electrical messages from your brain to the organ or tissue. If your muscles or any tissue do not get these electrical messages then that tissue or muscle dies.

The Muscles

There are many different muscles that attach to the spine. In this section we will talk about the most important muscles that contribute to your spine's function.

Can you feel the muscles in your back on either side of your lower spine? These muscles are called erector spinae. If you have ever gotten muscle spasms, these are the muscles going through the spasms. Underneath the erector spinae are smaller muscles that attach from one vertebra to the next. Underneath these are even smaller muscles that attach to the facet joints.

A major muscle in the front that is very important is the illio-psoas muscle. This is a big powerful muscle that is deep in your body that attaches directly to the front of the lumbar spine, goes across the hip joint, and attaches to the top of your femur (thigh bone).

Also in the front of your body are the abdominal muscles. These muscles are critical to the stability of your spine. They provide support and strength for your back. That is why abdominal exercises are so important in any back pain rehabilitation program.

Types and Causes of Back Pain

Millions of people each year suffer from lower back pain. The symptoms vary from mild to severe, and the effects can range from a slight nuisance to the inability to perform normal daily activities.

Back pain is real and can be debilitating. Some doctors that can't see the cause of your pain may think that you are exaggerating. If you experience this kind of treatment immediately find another doctor for a second opinion.

There are many misunderstanding about pain because doctors can not really test for pain. They could test for a fracture by doing an X-ray, or test for infection by doing some lab work. But pain is very subjective. What is painful for one person may seem like nothing for another. Everyone has a different pain tolerance.

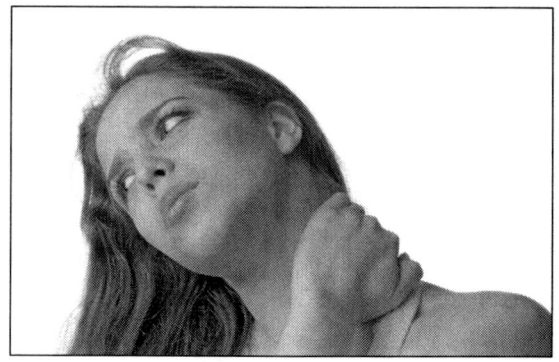

To add to the confusion, the cause of back pain is often difficult to figure out. So patients go through tests, and evaluations, and treatment after treatment, only to find that they still have the problem. By the time patients come to me, they have been just about everywhere. And pretty much had everything done to them.

Understanding where the pain is coming from is the first step to recovery.

Understanding Categories of Pain

There are three types of pain. It is important to understand these different types because treatment for each type is different.

1. **Acute pain.** Acute pain is pain that been happening for less than a four weeks. Usually it is related to tissue damage or trauma. This is the kind of pain that you experience when you have some injury like a broken leg or sprained ankle. The greater the injury, the greater the pain.

2. **Chronic pain.** Chronic pain is pain that has been going on for a long time, usually more than 12 weeks. It's the kind of pain that doesn't go away and for some reason the tissue is not able to properly heal. Chronic pain can originate from an injury that happened a long time ago or it could have been from some sort of repetitive stress. Most back pain suffers tend to fall into the chronic pain category.

3. **Recurrent acute pain, also know as intermittent pain.** This is the flare-up that happens over and over again.

The Need to Diagnose: Helpful or Harmful?

Finding out what is causing your pain is very important. Correct treatment always deals with removing the cause of your problem. Unfortunately patients go from diagnosis to diagnosis and from treatment to treatment without getting better. The reason I feel that this happens is because each diagnosis specifically targets one system in your body without looking at the whole person.

In this section we will discuss some of the common diagnoses for low-back pain. One word of warning while reading this section: do not get the medical student syndrome. This is when medical students read about different diseases and think they have the same symptoms. It's the saying a "little knowledge can be harmful."

After you read this section, you will know exactly what your doctor is talking about when he or she says something like sciatica, herniated disc, or degenerative disc disease. You will know appropriate questions to ask them to obtain the best treatments available for you.

Diagnosing Based Upon an Imaging Scan

Many doctors diagnose the cause of back pain just through some sort of imaging scan. The imaging scan is a great way to see what is happening on the inside but it is only one part of the solution. A complete workup would involve more than just a scan.

Also many times just because you see a herniated disc or arthritic changes in your

X-ray or MRI doesn't necessarily mean that the pain is coming from that specifically. In fact, your pain could be coming from an entirely different set of causes. If your doctor stops there and doesn't look at the whole picture your progress may be slow to zero.

Psychological and Emotional Factors

Psychological and emotional factors are critical in the role of back pain. The kind of stress you have, how long the stress has been part of your life, and the way your body is handling stress are all important factors of you losing your back pain. Can stress cause pain? Absolutely it can. Stress will dramatically change your physiology to the point where you may experience anything from flare-ups to depression to decreased immune response.

Your doctor should know the importance of emotional factors of your back pain. If he or she doesn't, you are probably not going to get the correct treatment. It is a fact that things like negative emotions or stress can cause and perpetuate many back pain cases. In later chapters you will learn to how to effectively deal with these stresses.

Emotional influences are so important to your overall picture that if your doctor does not consider it, the likelihood of you getting the appropriate care is low. If you feel that an emotional factor is involved with your back pain, then make sure you talk to your doctor about it. If your doctor does not seem interested or involved in this aspect, then it is time to find someone else who will treat you as a whole person, both mind and body.

Understanding the Deconditioning Syndrome

Deconditioning syndrome, also known as deactivation syndrome, occurs when you try to limit your movements or activities because of your back pain. This also happens when you rest too much. One thing that you have to remember is that "movement is life." Once you start limiting your movement the deconditioning syndrome will have a chance to set in.

Have you heard that bed rest is the worst thing for back pain? Well, believe it, it's true. As soon as you limit or avoid activity, deconditioning syndrome starts. By the way, some doctors still prescribe bed rest for back pain. Reducing activity will make your muscle imbalances worse. First of all, the lack of activity will weaken muscles, and decrease flexibility in your ligaments, tendons, and muscles. Your core stability muscles (the important core group of muscles) will suffer greatly for it. Decreased activity will also affect your mood, metabolism, and your heart.

An easy way to avoid deconditioning syndrome is to follow a core stability exercise program. A good program will start from where you are and slowly help you increase your strength and flexibility. The exercise program should not cause you any pain. In fact it should be relaxing.

Conditions That Cause Back Pain

The cause of back pain is very difficult to diagnose because it is rarely just physical. There are many other factors that contribute to back pain. One of the biggest factors is the relationship between mind and body.

In this section I am going to discuss some of the back pain diagnoses. You may have been labeled with some of them. Do not worry about that now because misdiagnosis is common when it comes to back pain.

I am going to go through many different types of conditions, some common and some rare. We will go through what the condition is, the common symptoms, how it is commonly diagnosed, and which treatment would work best for it.

Some rare but serious conditions like cauda equine syndrome, spinal tumor, or spinal infection requires immediate medical treatment. Your doctor will be able to diagnose these conditions quickly with proper testing.

Herniated Disc/Sciatica

Remember we discussed in the earlier chapter that vertebrae are stacked on top of each other and the disc lies between them. The disc acts as a cushion for your spine. The disc bulge or herniation usually occurs in phase two of degeneration. The bulge or herniation occurs because the disc has been getting less elastic, more unstable, weak and dehydrated. It becomes the weak link to your spine and any movement that compromises it will increase the likelihood of a possible bulge or herniation.

A bulge is where the disc wall is still intact, but the fluid inside, which is soft and gel-like, bulges out. Bulging discs can be seen easily in an MRI.

A herniation happens when the fluid gel-like substance inside the disc breaks through the outer wall of the disc called the annulus fibrosis. When the fluid inside the disc moves out of its normal space and breaks through the outer wall of the disc, it can irritate or press against a nerve, producing pain or other neurological symptoms.

One of the causes for sciatica can be a disc herniation. This can send pain down the leg or produce symptoms like burning, shooting pain. If the herniation presses on a motor nerve (nerve that control muscles), then you can experience muscle weakness, loss of balance, or cramps. Sciatica can also occur even if the nerve is not compressed but just irritated. Usually the pain is in the buttocks, back of the thigh or calf, and can even travel down the leg to the foot.

Most of the disc herniation occurs between the L4/L5 or L5/S1 segments. Actually more than 90 percent of herniations occur at those levels.

If your doctor thinks that your low back pain is coming from a herniated disc, then the following tips can help you get the right diagnosis.

TIP 1 **Make sure that your doctor does a full comprehensive exam.** This exam should be a full orthopedic and neurological examination. It should look at things like range of motion of your back, test for your hips, legs, and feet. The neurological portion of the exam should test how the nerves are working in the lower back, hips, legs, and feet. Your doctor should also test for muscle weakness, tightness, and any possible muscle imbalances. With a full comprehensive exam your doctor will be able to determine what further testing you will need. It could be anything from an MRI, CT scan, or more nerve tests.

TIP 2 **It is not always necessary to get an MRI or other sophisticated test to determine if you have a herniated disc.** After a careful physical exam, your doctor should be able to give a working diagnosis (a list of the most likely diagnosis for your condition). If your condition gets worse after a few treatments, or surgery is in consideration, then an Imaging scan would be necessary.

TIP 3 **Herniated discs do not always cause symptoms.** Just because your doctor finds a herniated disc on the MRI doesn't mean that particular herniation is causing your pain. The finding from a full orthopedic and neurological exam should correlate with the MRI to give the correct cause of your back pain.

If you just started to get symptoms of a disc herniation or a disc bulge, or you been having it for a less than a month, your doctor should find out which level the symptom is coming from and correlate that with any other testing you had done. You should start with conservative treatments such as chiropractic, physical therapy, exercises, better eating habits, and relaxation techniques. You can also try procedures like acupuncture, massage, or yoga.

A prognosis for disc herniation is very good. Surgery is rarely actually required. Most of my patients improve with a combination of chiropractic, disc decompression, core stability exercise, physical therapy, and stress-relief techniques. Some patients get better in a couple of weeks; some can take a few months of treatments. Everybody is different. What works for one person may not work for another. Again the reason to treat the whole person instead of just the low back pain.

Even if you do not recover 100 percent after three months don't panic. If you are improving even the slightest bit per day, you should continue with the treatment. You can also change the treatment around to see if that works better. Just because your pain is not totally gone does not mean you need surgery. Many doctors will recommend surgery because they just want to "try something." I will discuss later when a surgical recommendation is appropriate.

The Sprain-Strain Diagnosis

Sprain-strain means that there is either an injury to the muscle, ligament, or tendons of lower back. Usually the injury is due to a kind of major trauma such as sports injury, car accident, or a lifting injury, for example. The injury could also be due to some sort of minor trauma.

The thing most doctors miss about sprain-strain injury is that without proper treatment you can end up with permanent scar tissue either in the injured muscle, tendon, or ligament. Usually the affected area gets weak and is prone to further injury. A consistent treatment that strengthens the ligaments, tendons, and muscle is the best safeguard against recurring sprain-strain injuries. Resting and inactivity is one of the worst things you can do for a sprain-strain injury. You need make sure there is good blood circulation in those injured areas, and resting and babying it too much just won't do it.

Common symptoms of a sprain-strain injury are as follows:

- ❖ There are usually signs of pain, tightness, and spasms in the lower back area. The pain may be sharp and shooting or it could be a dull, aching pain. The pain could also build slowly and feel like a throbbing pain.
- ❖ There is increased tenderness around the affected area. The muscles on either side of your spine and your buttocks area can be tender to the touch.
- ❖ Pain may be elicited by movement. Bending side-to-side, or bending forward or backward may increase your pain.
- ❖ Back pain is evident right after you get up in the morning. Your lower back can be stiff and painful in the morning and then improve with movement and activity over the course of the day.

Diagnosis for sprain-strain is usually based on the exam and patient history. You can't actually see sprain-strain on an X-ray or blood test. If you have a sprain-strain injury due to some activity or movement being fearful of that movement can be a common reaction. Limiting any movement is not recommended because this can cause the start of deconditioning syndrome. Instead of limiting your activity and movement, try to rehabilitate and strengthen the injured area.

A typical treatment approach for a sprain-strain follows:

1. First, you should temporarily stop the activity and movement that cause pain, but you should continue some mild activity and gradually increase the activity to your normal level.

2. Use ice on the injured area to cool down the inflammation. You can get an ice pack or put some ice in a bag. Dampen a towel and wrap the towel around the bag. Do not have direct contact with the on your skin. You could leave the ice on the painful area for about 20 minutes.

3. If you can't stand the pain take a non-steroidal, anti-inflammatory medication.

4. Sprain-strain injuries may take three to four days to heal. Don't be in a rush; give your body a chance to heal.

5. Slowly return to your normal activity. Stretch and relax tight muscles and strengthen weak muscles.

Stress-related Back Pain

Based on my experience, stress can be the cause of many problems and conditions, including back pain. Other common symptoms stress can cause are insomnia, depression, anxiety, lethargy, and hormonal problems, just to name a few. Many doctors do not understand the stress-related back pain diagnosis. If you think that your back pain or the flare-ups are caused by stress, you want to make sure you let your doctor know about that.

Most doctors think that back pain is mainly a physical problem and so they focus on the physical causes. But if your back pain flares up because of emotional issues, or it becomes chronic because your body is not handling stress properly, dealing with these issues is critical for improvement. In later chapters we will talk about some new and very effective ways to handle stress.

Arthritis of the Spine

"Arthro" means joint and "it is" means inflammation. So arthritis is simply inflammation of the joint or joints in any part of the body. But what is important for your doctor to find out is what is actually causing the arthritis. Arthritis is typically diagnosed from X-rays or MRIs.

Degenerative Disc Disease and Lower Back Pain

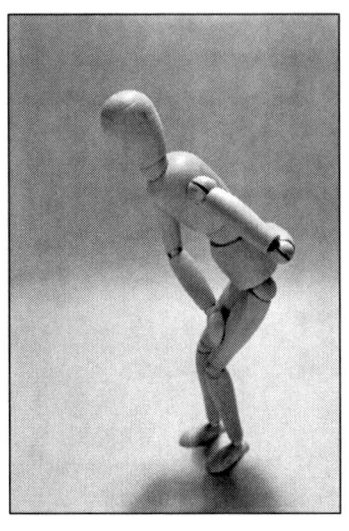

Why is it that lower back pain is such a widespread epidemic? To answer this question, it is necessary to examine the nature, causes, and symptoms of the most common source of lower back pain: degenerative disc disease, or DDD.

Although its name implies a serious disease that produces symptoms that worsen with time, the term degenerative disc disease is actually somewhat misleading. Before we examine what DDD is, it will be helpful to take a brief look at what it is not.

First, DDD is not strictly a "disease." Rather, it is a condition that signifies certain changes in the spinal discs. Second, while disc degeneration usually progresses over time as the name indicates, it does not necessary follow that the symptoms of degenerative disc disease worsen over time. In fact, in some cases, the symptoms actually lessen with time.

Even with this clarification, many medical providers disagree on the actual "pinpoint" definition of DDD. For the purposes of this book, however, we may establish the following general definition.

Is Degenerative Disc Disease Part of Aging?

Degenerative disc disease describes the changes that occur in the individual spinal discs as a person ages. Most medical practitioners agree that DDD is a normal part of aging, and many will say that it is, indeed, unavoidable.

The spinal column is composed of bony vertebrae separated by soft, spongy discs. These discs provide cushioning between the vertebrae and serve as shock absorbers within the spine. In addition, the discs allow for the natural movements of the spine such as bending, flexing, twisting, etc.

As individuals age, the spinal discs begin to lose fluid, flexibility, and absorption ability. The loss of fluid causes the discs to shrink and harden. To understand this more fully, imagine for a moment a basic kitchen sponge. When the sponge is wet, it is malleable, soft, and easily bent. As it dries, however, it shrivels up and becomes firm and more difficult to manipulate. The same is true of spinal discs. This hardening and consequent shrinking of the discs lessens the space between the vertebrae.

How The Spinal Disc Degenerates

As this occurs, the gel-like substance within the discs may begin to force out through tiny tears in the disc's outer layer. And this forced leakage may result in a bulging, ruptured, or even a broken disc.

All these activities occurring together cause the space between the vertebrae to shrink as the cushioning decreases, and this leads to spinal instability. In reaction to this, the body may begin to form bony growths, or spurs, and these bony growths put pressure on the nerve-rich spinal cord, causing pain and often impacting nerve function.

Symptoms of Degenerative Disc Disease

Despite the serious-sounding nature of degenerative disc disease, not everyone who has it experiences symptoms. In fact, many people with DDD have no pain at all. For those who do present symptoms of DDD, these symptoms may vary depending upon which portion of the spine is most severely affected.

Degenerative disc disease most often impacts the lower or lumbar spinal region or the neck or cervical region. Lumbar degenerative disc disease may cause back, leg, or buttocks pain, while cervical degenerative disc disease may result in pain in the neck or arm. In some cases, DDD is characterized by numbness or a tingling sensation in the arms or legs, and movements such as twisting, bending over, or reaching upward may exacerbate DDD pain.

While the onset of DDD may be triggered by a trauma, such as an automobile accident, major or minor fall, or even an everyday activity like bending over to lift an object, in some instances degenerative disc disease may begin without a specific trigger.

Although degenerative disc disease is considered a side-effect of aging, some people begin to experience the symptoms of DDD in their thirties, and oftentimes this sparks concern that the condition will worsen over time, eventually leading to an extreme debilitating condition. History, however, shows otherwise. While the disc degeneration may be progressive, the pain, while it occasionally can seem to be worsening, usually is not progressive over the long-term.

Diagnosing DDD

Diagnosing degenerative disc disease is usually accomplished through a complete physical examination in which the doctor reviews complaints of pain as well as tests for flexibility, range of motion, reflexes, and muscle strength. The examination will usually include X-rays to detect a narrowing of the spinal column and/or the presence of bone spurs. Additionally, a CT scan and/or an MRI may also be ordered to evaluate more fully the spinal column and its surrounding materials.

Treatment of DDD

If the doctor determines that the diagnosis is indeed degenerative disc disease, treatment may include correcting muscle imbalances, chiropractic adjustments, and non-steroidal anti-inflammatory drugs coupled with physical therapy. In very rare instances, surgery may be necessary.

While degenerative disc disease is one of the most common causes of back pain, it does not have to be a debilitating condition. With proper diagnosis and treatment, a person with DDD can continue to live an active and fulfilling life.

The Face of Facet Syndrome

Chances are you know someone who has been in a "fender bender." Perhaps you have even found yourself in this unpleasant situation. It is quite common for individuals who have been in automobile accidents ranging from minor to severe to complain of the common injury known as "whiplash."

What we call whiplash, however, could actually be indicative of a medical condition known as facet syndrome, and while whiplash is a major cause of facet syndrome, it is by no means the only cause. We are going to go over the definition, causes, and symptoms of facet syndrome.

What Is a Facet Joint?

By way providing a foundation for exploring facet syndrome, however, it is important to understand what the facet joints are, and to do this, we must take a look at the composition of the spine.

Each movable segment of the spine is comprised of three parts: the vertebra, the facet joint, and the intervertebral disc. The vertebra is the actual bony portion of the spine, the intervertebral discs are the cushioning discs between each vertebra, and the facet joints are small joints that are between and behind adjacent vertebrae and which act as stabilizers. While it is important that the spine be flexible enough to bend, twist, stretch, etc., it is equally vital that it remains stable while doing so, and the facet joints make this possible.

Facet joints are present at every vertebral level except for the top, and they provide twisting stability particularly in the cervical (neck) and lumbar (lower back) areas. The facet joints function and are positioned as follows:

At each spinal level, the facet joint is angled in such a way as to provide the necessary range of motion for that area while preventing vertebral slippage. The joints are attached on both sides of the backside of each vertebra, with their faces positioned either forwards or to the side. These faces reach downward to meet the upward facing joints on the vertebra below.

As motion occurs, the joints slide over each other, yet because the sliding surfaces are protected by moist cartilage and because a lubricant surrounds each joint, the natural sliding should not irritate the joint. The sack, which supplies the lubricant, however, is full of nerve fibers so in the event of irritation, a warning signal can be sent to the brain.

Because the back is constantly in motion due to everyday activities such as bending, reaching, lifting, and twisting, the wear and tear of daily movement often takes its toll on the facet joints. Cartilage can thin out; bone spurs can appear, and joints can become enlarged. This inflammation of the joint, characterized as arthritic, can produce back pain, particularly during motion, and this pain is termed "facet joint disease" or "facet joint syndrome." Simply stated, then, facet syndrome is the irritation of the facet joints.

Causes of Facet Syndrome

Various factors ranging from one-time injury to gradual weakening and chronic stress can lead to the onset of facet syndrome. Among the most common causes, however, are whiplash and certain athletic injuries most often occurring in activities, such as gymnastics, which require significant neck or spine extension.

Estimates show that as many as 90% of adults will experience facet joint syndrome at some point in their lives, and, interestingly, joint syndrome is the most common cause of disability in individuals under the age of 45. Moreover, facet joint syndrome has been identified as the second-leading reason for visits to primary care physicians and the leading reason people seek the care of orthopedic surgeons and neurosurgeons.

Symptoms of Facet Syndrome

The symptoms of facet syndrome are not unique to the condition and, particularly because of this, it is important that a healthcare professional perform a thorough evaluation to determine if the source of back pain is actually facet joint syndrome or if it is another, potentially more serious condition.

Generally, however, symptoms that are associated with facet syndrome include the following:

- Local tenderness on one or more of the facet joint areas
- Some loss of spinal muscle flexibility
- Diffused pain over the buttocks and, at times, the posterolateral thigh (It should be noted that pain which extends below the knee or into the foot or pain that is present in the front of the thigh is rarely associated with facet syndrome is often caused instead by disc herniation.)
- Pain which worsens with back hyperextension
- Pain which worsens when a position is held for any length of time
- Loss of curvature in the lower back
- Headaches
- Neck pain
- Loss of neck movement
- Pain that radiates into the upper back (Again, however, pain which extends into the front or down the arm and into the fingers may be indicative of a herniated disc.)

As with any back pain or discomfort, it is important to obtain a professional diagnosis to determine its cause. The appropriate treatment can then be prescribed and the journey to restored health begins.

Understanding the Reality of Stress-related Back Pain

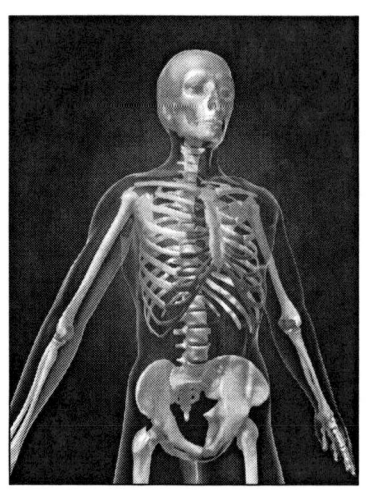

Back pain is a silent epidemic, affecting millions of people of all ages and often hindering their ability to live life to the fullest. Numerous medical conditions and abnormalities can contribute to back pain, including direct injury, degenerative disorders, arthritis, tumors, or other bone or spinal diseases.

Aside from the medical factors, however, there is one type of back pain that, while causing symptoms of real physical discomfort, is in reality a psychosomatic or psycho-physiological disorder. This is tension myositis syndrome (TMS) or, more commonly termed, stress-related back pain.

For some time, the medical community has generally acknowledged that physical conditions can be affected by psychological factors. The official diagnosis of stress-related back pain, however, recognizes that emotional and psychological factors not only affect back pain, but they may be the primary cause of it.

History of Stress-related Back Pain

Although the idea of stress-related back pain has a history dating back to the 1820s, the concept has more recently been popularized and promoted by physician and New York University professor of physical medicine and rehabilitation Dr. John Sarno.

Psychologist and spine specialist Dr. William Deardorff writes that at its origin in the nineteenth century, what we today would call stress-related back pain was identified as "spinal irritation." Rather than being supported by medical evidence, the diagnosis of spinal irritation was often given when symptoms were vague and an official diagnosis could not be determined.

In his book *From Paralysis to Fatigue: A History of Psychosomatic Illness in the Modern Era,* Dr. Edward Shorter indicates that physicians in the 1900s might have diagnosed a patient with spinal irritation as a sort of "face-saving" mechanism to avoid resorting to openly psychological and emotional diagnoses. Even with this diagnostic conclusion, however, early doctors continued to prescribe physical treatments to address the elusive problem.

Returning to the present, Dr. Sarno has concluded that of the countless back pain cases being treated within the medical community today, the majority should actually be diagnosed as stress-related. Specifically, Dr. Sarno's theory of TMS can be summarized as follows:

- Back pain is brought on not by medical, mechanical, or physical causes but rather by psychological factors including feelings, personality tendencies, and even unconscious emotional or other issues.
- Certain emotions and personality types and traits contribute most to stress-related back pain.
- When these personality traits combine with stress-filled situations in life, back pain ensues.
- Despite the reality of the pain, its source is not always readily identifiable.

Are You Predisposed to Stress-related Back Pain?

While stress-related back pain can affect anyone, Dr. Sarno holds that the emotions that are often related to it are unconscious anger and rage. Moreover, the following personality traits place individuals at a higher risk of developing TMS:

- ❖ Type A personality
- ❖ High sense of responsibility
- ❖ Perfectionistic tendencies
- ❖ Compulsive nature
- ❖ Self-critical
- ❖ Self-disciplined
- ❖ Self-motivated
- ❖ Inwardly driven to succeed

Individuals with one or more of these tendencies may be likely unconsciously to disregard emotional tension. The tension, however, continues to affect the body and can adversely impact the nervous system. Changes in the system may display as constriction of blood vessels and subsequent reduction in blood flow to important nerves, tissues, and muscles of the body. These unseen alterations can produce the noticeable effects of pain, tension, and even muscle spasms.

Unfortunately, the presence of pain then contributes to increased tension, causing increased pain, until patients may find themselves unable to perform tasks ranging from overt physical activity to normal daily movements.

How to Identify Stress-related Back Pain

Despite its seemingly elusive nature, stress-related back pain can be correctly identified. Patients should not assume, however, that back pain is stress-related without obtaining a professional diagnosis, as it is important to rule out the presence of other serious medical conditions.

Diagnosing stress-related back pain usually involves a thorough physical examination and medical history review. Specifically, doctors may look for the following:

- ❖ Various muscle aches
- ❖ Back or neck pain
- ❖ Pain in general movement
- ❖ Fatigue and sleep difficulties

Beating Stress-related Back Pain

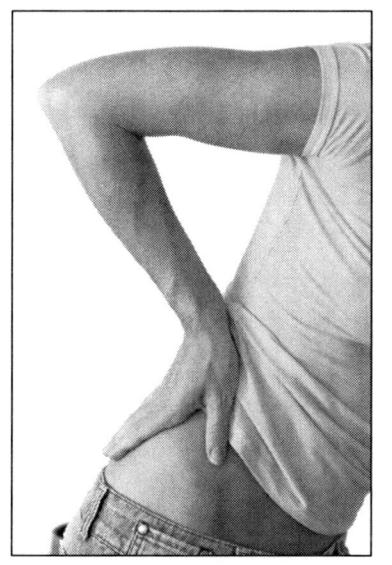

Once a diagnosis of TMS is accurately reached, several treatment options are available. Those following Dr. Sarno's theory will prescribe treatment that addresses psychological and emotional factors, particularly repressed emotions. Others will adapt a broader approach that takes into account physical, emotional, cognitive, and environmental issues that may be causing or impacting the pain.

Even though treatment is available, the ideal situation is to prevent stress-related back pain from impacting your life. While it is impossible to eliminate all sources of stress, it is certainly possible to develop habits to minimize the negative impact of stress. One of the best ways to do this is to develop a healthy lifestyle, which includes regular physical activity. Exercise increases blood flow and air circulation throughout the body, and it is an effective mechanism for reducing stress. In addition, seek to minimize or eliminate sources of stress both at work and at home. For the person with perfectionist tendencies, self-established deadlines and standards can create artificial sources of stress. Certainly, real deadlines do exist, but be aware when stressful situations are created internally rather than externally, and be willing to reevaluate self-imposed demands.

Finally, take time to pause in your daily activity to simply relax for a few moments. Take a walk outside, write your thoughts down on paper, or chat with a friend.

Although stress will always be a part of natural life, you can reduce your risk of developing stress-related back pain by working to minimize it.

Arachnoiditis: Symptoms, Causes, and Treatment Options

In 1990, Hollywood made arachnophobia — the fear of spiders — a household word. Frightening as this phobia is, there is another "arachno" in existence that is far more debilitating and far less known. It is arachnoiditis, and while it has nothing to do with the fear of insects, it can be just as paralyzing.

What Is Arachnoiditis?

Simply stated, arachnoiditis is a medical condition caused by an inflammation of the arachnoid lining around the brain and spinal cord. The brain and spinal cord are protected, surrounded, and cushioned by three membranes. The first membrane, the dura mater, is tough and fibrous in consistency. As the outermost of the three membranes, the dura mater lines the inner surface of the skull.

Next to the dura mater is the arachnoid membrane. This membrane has been defined as "delicate," and it forms the middle of the three membranes. The innermost membrane, lying next to the arachnoid, is the pia mater. This vascular membrane is the closest of the three to the brain and spinal cord.

In addition to these three membranes, a layer of cerebrospinal fluid (CSF) occupies the subarachnoid space between the arachnoid membrane and the pia mater. This CSF acts as a shock absorber.

Arachnoiditis is the condition characterized by inflammation of this middle, arachnoid layer. Other terms used for arachnoiditis, although less commonly, are arachnitis, chronic adhesive arachnoiditis (CAA), and spinal fibrosis.

Symptoms of Arachnoiditis

The most prevalent symptoms of arachnoiditis are chronic pain in the lower back, lower limbs, or, at times, in the entire body. Aside from these dominant symptoms, however, several other symptoms may also surface with arachnoiditis. According to the late Dr. Edgar G. Dawson, expert spine surgeon and authority in the field of orthopedic surgery, additional symptoms of arachnoiditis may include the following:

- ❖ Tingling, numbness, or weakness in the legs
- ❖ Sensory sensations akin to insects crawling on the skin or water trickling down over the skin/legs
- ❖ Severe shooting pain resembling that from an electric shock
- ❖ Muscle cramps, spasms, or uncontrollable twitching
- ❖ Bladder, bowel, and/or sexual dysfunction

Arachnoiditis may also cause a burning or stinging sensation in the lower back or legs and, in severe cases, paralysis of the lower limbs.

What Causes Arachnoiditis?

As mentioned, arachnoiditis is caused by the inflammation of the arachnoid membrane. As outlined by the National Institute of Neurological Disorders and Stroke, part of the US National Institutes of Health, this inflammation can be triggered by numerous factors, including the following:

- ❖ Chemical irritation
- ❖ Infection from bacteria or viruses
- ❖ Direct injury to the spine
- ❖ Chronic compression of spinal nerves
- ❖ Complications from spinal surgery
- ❖ Complications from other invasive spinal procedures

Inflammation from any of these causes can result in scarring and the formation of scar tissue and adhesions. These can lead to a sort of fusion, "sticking together," of the spinal nerves. It is when this fusion impinges upon normal nerve function that the symptoms of tingling and stinging can occur.

It should be noted here, however, that while arachnoiditis most often impacts the nerves which affect the lower back and legs, the condition has no strict pattern of symptoms, and even something as seemingly unrelated as a skin rash can be related to arachnoiditis.

Diagnosis of Arachnoiditis

The most accurate means of diagnosis arachnoiditis is through the use of a positive computed tomography (CT) or magnetic resonance imaging (MRI) scan, coupled with the presence of one or more symptoms. Even with these methods, however, if the condition is in the early stages, imaging tests may return negative results, becoming more positive only as the condition worsens. To detect arachnoiditis in its early stages, certain cell and protein tests may prove helpful. However, health experts indicate that there are cases in which an authoritative diagnosis unfortunately may not be possible.

How to Treat Arachnoiditis

There is currently no cure for arachnoiditis, and treatment presently remains aimed at reducing inflammation and alleviating pain in patients suffering from the disorder. Medications prescribed in the treatment process may include both steroidal and non-steroidal anti-inflammatories as well as other narcotic and non-narcotic pain medications.

In addition to these, other treatment options include steroid injections, transcutaneous electrical nerve stimulation (TENS), alternative medical treatments, or topical analgesics. One newer treatment for alleviating pain is direct spinal cord stimulation. In this process, electrodes are placed underneath the skin and directly on the affected nerve roots. A surgically placed battery-powered unit supplies currents through these electrodes in order to stop pain signals and thus alleviate pain symptoms.

A more invasive and more controversial treatment involves direct surgery to remove the affected tissue at the location of inflammation. The surgical option may also entail removing a small piece of vertebrae and/or scar tissue in the affected area. However, this option is not widely accepted since surgery results in the development of even more scar tissues and further exposes the spinal cord to irritation. Furthermore, while surgery may provide temporary relief, long-term studies have often shown regression over a time span of several years.

Unfortunately, the prognosis for curing arachnoiditis is poor. While researchers continue to search for a cure, treatment options for patients currently suffering from the condition should focus on pain alleviation so they may continue to live productive lives.

Identification, Causes, and Diagnosis of "Slipped Disc"

We are all familiar with the term "slipped disc," but chances are that few of us have ever heard of isthmic spondylolisthesis. This tongue-twister word is actually the medical term for a slipped disk, and among the myriad causes of back pain, it is among the most common in adolescents. Yet despite its widespread nature, it is hardly a household word. Its very prevalence, however, issues a mandate that we more fully understand this condition, including what causes it, how it presents itself, and the tests necessary to diagnose it.

Following is a brief overview of spondylolisthesis, including an examination of its closely related and contributing condition, spondylolysis.

What is a Slipped Disc?

Technically speaking, the term spondylolisthesis comes from the Latin and means "slipped vertebral body." Spondylolisthesis is a condition in which all or part of a vertebra in the spine slips forward onto another vertebra. The most common type of spondylolisthesis is isthmic spondylolisthesis, and it often occurs in children as young as 5 to 8 years of age although it is also commonly seen in adolescents ages 10 to 15. Approximately 5% of the population will experience isthmic spondylolisthesis.

Contrasted with this, spondylolysis is a fracture or a defect that occurs in the pars interarticularis, or meeting point of the vertebra between two facet joints. Spondylolysis acts similarly to a loose hinge and can lead to instability in the vertebral column. Spondylolysis is the most common cause of isthmic spondylolisthesis. While the terms are sometimes used interchangeably, it is incorrect to do so as each indicates a separate condition.

Causes of Slipped Disc

Spondylolysis is often caused by repeated extension and rotation of the back. These activities result in the application of increased force in the lumbar spine and increased pressures to the facet joints. The pars interarticularis is called upon to bear the force of the increased pressure. Because the pars interarticularis is small, however, it is often unable to sustain itself under repeated force and pressure. As a result, a stress fracture — or spondylolysis — will develop.

As it is often caused by activities involving repeated back extension, spondylolysis is commonly seen in athletes who participate in sports such as gymnastics, javelin throwing, rowing, boxing, weightlifting, high jump, diving, and wrestling.

When continually subjected to ongoing stress, spondylolysis can lead to spondylolisthesis, or a slipped vertebra. As the muscles and ligaments of the vertebral column strive to maintain the structure of the spinal column, the stress may eventually prove too much, and one or more vertebrae can slide forward. This slippage can result in a pinched nerve and consequent pain.

While children and adolescents involved in certain athletic activities are at an increased risk for developing spondylolysis and spondylolisthesis, these conditions can also occur in adults. When they do, however, they are often brought on by non-athletic causes, including disc and facet joint degeneration and other factors.

How to Diagnose Slipped Disc

To diagnose spondylolysis and spondylolisthesis, doctors may utilize several techniques including some or all of the following:

- ❖ **X-rays** While X-rays may be helpful in detecting vertebral cracks or slippages, they are not fool-proof.

- ❖ **CAT scan** A more accurate method of detecting cracks in bones, a CAT scan can be a useful diagnostic tool.

- ❖ **MRI** An MRI allows a doctor to see the relationships between the various spinal structures, thus facilitating detection of a vertebra slippage.

- ❖ **Michelis' test** Also called the one-legged hyperextension maneuver, this test positions the patient on one leg so that the lumbar spine is hyperextended. The patient then repeats this position on the opposite side. The presence of pain with the maneuver may indicate spondylolysis.

In addition to tests to detect the presence of spondylolysis and/or spondylolisthesis, a doctor will also perform tests to rule out other problems which may cause back pain, such as diabetes, tumors, or cancer.

Once an accurate diagnosis is reached, several treatment options exist, and the choice of which option to pursue may depend upon the nature and severity of the condition. Oftentimes, a doctor will recommend activity restrictions, particularly in patients involved in athletics or other physical activities. If spondylolysis has not yet progressed to spondylolisthesis, however, activity restriction may not always be required.

In adults showing symptoms of spondylolisthesis, a doctor may advise them to refrain from intense physical activity and physically demanding jobs. Additionally, a doctor may prescribe anti-inflammatory medications to reduce swelling and pain-relieving medications to minimize discomfort. In many cases, chiropractic adjustments with specific back-strengthening exercises work very well for this condition.

Although spondylolysis will not always lead to spondylolisthesis, it is important that anyone, whether young or old, who is experiencing symptoms which may be indicative of either one of these conditions seek medical treatment immediately. If spondylolysis alone is present, steps can be taken to prevent the further injury of spondylolisthesis and, in cases in which spondylolisthesis has already occurred, a doctor can offer options to alleviate the pain and treat this condition.

Coccydynia: The *REAL* Pain in the Tailbone

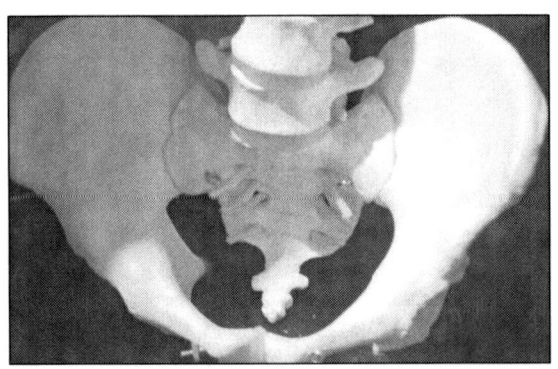

For those who have never experienced coccydynia, the term "pain in the rear" is merely an expression easily tossed into conversation. But for the person who suffers from coccydynia, this flippant term is all too serious.

What exactly is coccydynia? What are the causes and symptoms? How can someone determine if he or she suffers from it? Who is at risk for this condition, and is it treatable? For answers to these questions and more, read on.

What is Coccydynia?

Coccydynia is defined as pain in the coccyx. Commonly known as the tailbone, the coccyx is the small, triangular-shaped bone at the base of the spine, and it is formed by the fusion of several — usually four — vertebrae. Alternate names for coccydynia include coccygodynia, coccygeal pain, and coccyx pain.

Symptoms of Coccydynia

Coccydynia often produces symptoms as simple as pain or soreness in the tailbone area, particularly at the very base of the spine. The pain is often persistent, localized, and more acutely felt when sitting. Coccydynia also causes tenderness in the area of the coccyx and can produce pain that worsens due to constipation or during a bowel movement.

What Causes Coccydynia?

Oftentimes, coccydynia is caused by a specific injury, such as a fall, or in women by childbirth. Certain activities, however, can also trigger the onset of this condition. For example, pressure-inducing activities, such as bicycling and horseback riding, which place direct pressure on the coccyx, may bring on coccydynia.

In rare instances, other medical conditions including an undiagnosed sacrococcygeal teratoma, or SCT, may cause coccydynia. An SCT is a tumor that can be present in newborns and is found at the coccyx. While SCT is considered a birth defect, it is usually curable through surgery following birth. This type of tumor is more common in females than in males, and, if left undiagnosed, it can lead to coccydynia. In addition to SCT, other tumors in the tailbone area may cause coccydynia, although this is rare. More likely, this painful condition is the result of a fall or childbirth.

Important Tips for Diagnosing Coccydynia

In diagnosing coccydynia, it is important that the healthcare provider be well-versed in the condition, as there also exist other causes of tailbone pain, which, while producing symptoms similar to coccydynia, should not be diagnosed as such. These include a fractured bone, sciatica (a pinched or irritated nerve root in the lower spine), infection, or a pilonidal cyst (a skin infection near the tailbone).

Usually, coccydynia can be diagnosed through an evaluation of symptoms alone, including an examination to determine the presence of local tenderness. To rule out the presence of other conditions, however, a healthcare provider may perform additional examination and/or testing. These may include examination to detect a localized rash, which might indicate the presence of shingles, or a CAT scan or MRI to exclude the possibility of a more serious bone or tissue disorder.

How to Treat Coccydynia

Once a diagnosis of coccydynia has been accurately reached, there are several treatment options available, most of which are simple, at-home, remedies aimed at alleviating pain and assisting in recovery.

Patients diagnosed with coccydynia will usually be advised to use padded seats or a padded seating accessory such as a donut pillow and to refrain from remaining seated for extended periods of time. Patients should plan to rest the area in order to avoid the threat of re-injury. In certain instances, anti-inflammatory medications or doctor-approved pain relievers may help to alleviate the symptoms present with coccydynia. In addition, if tailbone pain becomes worse with bowel movements, stool softeners and a diet rich in fiber may be recommended to help alleviate this discomfort.

In many cases, these simple treatment options will be sufficient to restore health and wellbeing to the coccyx. However, if the pain persists or worsens, more aggressive doctor-administered treatments may be required. It is important to note that there are specific chiropractic techniques that can relieve pressure and pain from the coccyx.

Doctors treating patients with persistent coccydynia may recommend cortisone injections. Cortisone (a type of corticosteroid) is a strong anti-inflammatory medication. While not a pain reliever in and of itself, cortisone often alleviates pain through reducing inflammation.

Patients requiring cortisone injections to treat coccydynia will receive these injections in the doctor's office, and many patients find that this simple treatment is sufficient to relieve their tailbone pain.

In extreme cases of coccydynia in which neither home treatment nor cortisone injections adequately alleviate pain and discomfort, a physician may recommend a coccygectomy, or surgical removal of the coccyx. In the early 1900s, this extreme treatment was more common than it is today as coccydynia was often the diagnosis given to most lower back pain. As health and medical research has advanced, however, it is now known that coccydynia, while a viable medical condition, causes only a small percentage of lower back pain conditions.

Coccydynia can be a very painful condition that impinges upon normal, day-to-day activities. However, with rest and simple home treatments, the pain of coccydynia can often be alleviated and natural healing can usually occur.

Identifying and Understanding Symptoms and Warning Signs of Spinal Fractures

Common understanding of skeletal fractures holds that they occur as a direct result of sudden trauma, such as a fall, automobile accident, or other blunt-force impact. While this assumption is true for a wide variety of fractures, it is not always a reliable conclusion when it comes to spinal or vertebral fractures. Indeed, any number of causes may result in a spinal fracture.

Unfortunately, because the symptoms of spinal fractures are not always as acute as they often are with other skeletal fractures, it is possible for spinal fractures to remain undiagnosed and, consequently, untreated. To maintain back health and overall physical health, it is important to understand the causes of vertebral fractures and to recognize possible warning signs that may indicate a condition which requires treatment.

The Spinal Column

The spinal column is comprised of thirty-three bones, or vertebrae, which constitute the main support structure of the body. Together, these vertebrae form the spinal canal which protects the spinal cord, the body's sensitive nerve hub through which messages are relayed from the brain to the rest of the body. Openings between the vertebrae allow spinal nerves to branch out from the spinal cord to carry these messages throughout the body. Hence, the vertebral column performs the two key functions of structural support and nerve protection. It is easy to understand, then, the importance of maintaining vertebral health and the serious negative impact spinal fractures can have on overall body functioning.

Overview of Spinal Fractures

While spinal fractures can occur at any location along the spinal column, the majority of fractures occur in the lower back. In fact, over 60% of spinal fractures occur in this area, with between 5 and 10% occurring in the cervical, or neck, area.

In studying spinal fractures, experts have classified them according to three categories: fractures, dislocations, and fracture-dislocations.

Fractures occur when a bone breaks due to excessive pressure. A **compression fracture** in the back can result from sudden and strong downward force exerted upon the spinal column or from progressive weakening of the bones through osteoporosis or other diseases.

Dislocations signify vertebrae coming out of proper alignment. Dislocation may result from the stretching or tearing of ligaments and/or discs between vertebrae. A common cause of spinal dislocation would be whiplash during an automobile accident.

Fracture-dislocations result from a combination of the above two scenarios and are the most harmful of spinal fractures.

Causes of Spinal Fractures

Causes of spinal fractures can vary greatly; however, the most common causes include the following:

- ❖ Car accidents, accounting for approximately 45% of spinal fractures
- ❖ Falls, accounting for approximately 20%
- ❖ Athletics, accounting for approximately 15%
- ❖ Violent acts, including gunshots, accounting for approximately 15%
- ❖ Miscellaneous activities, accounting for approximately 5%

In addition, weakening of the bones due to diseases such as osteoporosis can also contribute to spinal fractures, particularly in older women. The extent of injury from these fractures can range from minor to severe.

Warning Signs of Spinal Fractures

Spinal fractures are not always immediately noticeable. In fact, a person may continue for months or even years without recognizing he or **she** has a spinal fracture. There are several warning signs that should not be ignored as **they** may indicate the presence of a spinal fracture requiring attention.

Signs that might warn of spinal fracture may include the following:

- ❖ Back or neck pain
- ❖ Numbness or tingling sensations
- ❖ Muscle spasms
- ❖ Weakness
- ❖ Changes in bowel/bladder habits
- ❖ Partial or complete paralysis

While common conception defines a spinal fracture as a serious injury — and, indeed, it can be — symptoms do not always appear serious. For this reason, it is particularly important to pay attention to seemingly insignificant symptoms and to report them to a professional healthcare provider. Indeed, spinal fractures may begin as little more than a backache. This is particularly true of compression fractures, which occur in women (or men) with osteoporosis. At-risk populations should be especially alert to these warning signs for compression fractures:

- ❖ Back pain that worsens when standing or walking
- ❖ Loss of height
- ❖ Spine deformity, such as a curved or hunched shape
- ❖ Severe and sudden back pain

Additionally, with multiple compression fractures, internal organs can be affected, and the injured person may experience any or all of the following:

- ❖ Trouble breathing, as the lungs are impacted by a severely compressed spine
- ❖ Stomach problems, including digestive complaints resulting from a compressed stomach
- ❖ Hip pain caused by the ribs and hip bones rubbing together as a result of a compressed spine

Diagnosis of Spinal Fracture

Diagnosing spinal fractures can be done using any one or more of several methods.

- ❖ **X-rays** to examine vertebrae to detect bone fractures. Flexion and extension X-rays may also be used to uncover any unusual vertebral movement
- ❖ **CT scans** to view the spinal column layer by layer to detect any abnormalities. The CT scan may also include dye injection to make visible any variations in bone structure.
- ❖ **MRIs** to provide a three-dimensional view of the spine. Like a CT scan, an MRI can also be performed using a dyeing agent. MRIs are particularly useful for examining ligament and disc injuries.

While spinal injuries can be serious, many spinal fractures are treatable. Understanding their causes and symptoms will empower at-risk individuals to recognize warning signs and take the necessary steps to detect and treat spinal fractures.

Subluxation: The Silent Killer

Nearly everyone has experienced back discomfort at one point or another. Discomfort can range from the feeling that something is simply "out of line" to persistent pain that hinders the accomplishment of required jobs and tasks.

While we may offhandedly refer to the pain we feel as simply "back pain" or as having something "out of whack," this common discomfort that affects millions of people has a name. And since knowledge is power, understanding the nature, causes, and treatments of this silent disease is the first step in combating back pain for good.

Subluxation Defined

The medical term for this widespread "out of whack" feeling is **subluxation**. In Latin "sub" means less than, and "luction" means dislocation. Simply stated, subluxation is the condition that exists when a joint or organ is partially dislocated from its normal position. According to the World Health Organization (WHO), subluxation is deemed a "significant structural displacement" noticeable enough to be detected through static imaging studies, i.e. X-rays.

Subluxation can affect a number of joints throughout the body, including the elbow, shoulder, fingers, and kneecaps. For the purpose of this article, however, focus will be placed upon subluxation as it affects the back and spinal column.

This type of subluxation, also termed **vertebral subluxation**, refers to a common condition in which a vertebra in the spinal column moves or slips out of alignment with one or both of its adjacent vertebrae. When this occurs, the out-of-place vertebra places undue pressure on the nerve, thus causing discomfort, pain, and confusing nerve signals.

Your Nervous System

To understand this fully, it is worthwhile to review briefly the basic workings of the human nervous system.

From the central hub of the brain, the nervous system controls all aspects of the body's functioning. Electrical impulses issued from the master control center (a.k.a., the brain) travel along the spinal cord and to the nerves that branch off from the spinal cord to various parts of the body. These nerves escape the spinal column through small openings between the vertebrae.

When vertebrae are in their proper positions, the impulses can travel freely through the nerves. If a vertebra slips or becomes dislodged due to injury, strain, or any other cause, the opening or passageway for the nerves can become constricted, and as pressure is placed on the nerves, the brain's electronic impulse messages may become hindered or distorted. Depending upon the extent of the vertebral dislocation and consequent nerve pressure, the effects of this distortion in the body can become noticeable and painful.

Symptoms of Subluxation

Symptoms of subluxation can vary from the obvious to the less pronounced, and at times the only way to accurately detect subluxation will be through professional examination. When symptoms are noticeable, patients may experience any one or more of the following:

❖ Pain in various parts of the body

❖ Soreness

❖ Digestive troubles

❖ Feelings of weakness

❖ Other health irregularities

Causes of Subluxation

While subluxation can be caused by any number of factors, one of the most common causes of vertebral subluxation is an automobile accident. The sudden trauma to the spinal column, commonly referred to as whiplash, can often result in vertebral subluxation. Other activities can also cause this discomforting condition. These include athletic participation, lifting heavy objects, and even sitting for extended periods of time.

How to Diagnose Subluxation

To determine if the root cause of any of these symptoms is subluxation, a healthcare provider may rely on one or more of several diagnosing options. For serious injuries, such as those brought on by automobile accidents or athletic activities, diagnostic imaging (i.e., X-rays, MRIs, CT scans, etc.) may detect the presence of subluxation.

Less noticeable instances of subluxation are best located through professional examination by a trained chiropractor. A skilled chiropractor will often be able to detect subluxations through a hands-on examination of the spinal column and other joints. During the examination, a chiropractor will look for any signs of abnormal functioning including joint movement that is either too limited or too liberal, the presence of pain, and even uneven limb length.

Proper Treatment for Subluxation

Treatment of subluxation often involves chiropractic adjustment to return vertebrae to healthy position and relieve pressure on the nerves. This adjustment is usually performed manually, although at times hand-held chiropractic instruments may also be utilized. It should be noted that chiropractors are the only healthcare professionals with the benefit of years of training in accurately correcting subluxation, and the vast majority of adjustments in the United States are performed by doctors of chiropractic. In instances of more serious injury in which treatment other than adjustment is required, a professional chiropractor will recognize the same and make further recommendations and consultation.

Prognosis

Subluxation is often called "the silent killer" because it can occur undetected. Depending on the severity of the subluxation and the area affected, the body may not always send out warnings of irregular functioning. In cases in which subluxation remains undetected, organ damage may occur. Doctors of chiropractic are specifically trained and skilled in detecting subluxations, and when they are detected, chiropractic care can usually remedy them and return the body to a healthy alignment.

Lumbar Spinal Stenosis: Causes, Symptoms, and Diagnosis

The human body is a magnificently intricate creation, and forming the main support structure of the body is the all-important spinal column. The skeletal structure of the spine is made up of the bony vertebrae, with each individual vertebra separated from its neighbor by a spongy disc. Together, the vertebrae form a column which supports the body. As a whole, the spinal column bears up approximately half of the total weight of the body, while muscles support the other half.

An injury or abnormality in any part of the spinal column may cause pain and discomfort and in some cases may lead to more serious conditions such as partial or complete paralysis. Unfortunately, back pain and discomfort is all too common, and among the most common type of back pain from which individuals suffer is lower, or lumbar, back pain. In many cases, this pain is the result of a condition known as lumbar spinal stenosis.

What Is Spinal Stenosis?

Before examining lumbar spinal stenosis in greater detail, it is helpful to review very briefly the general anatomy of the spine. While the spine forms one column, it is subdivided into three specific regions: the cervical spine, the thoracic spine, and the lumbar spine. The cervical spine, or neck area, contains seven vertebral segments. The thoracic spine, or lung area/upper back, is comprised of the next twelve vertebrae. Because these bones are firmly attached to the ribs and sternum, they present a lesser risk for injury than their lower counterparts. Finally, the bottom five vertebrae form the lumbar spine, or lower back. It is this area that bears the greatest percentage of the body's weight.

Spinal stenosis is the condition characterized by the narrowing of the spinal canal resulting from bone or tissue growth. This growth causes the size of the spinal canal opening to decrease, thus placing pressure on the spinal nerves and, at times, even on the spinal cord. Although spinal stenosis can occur in the neck, lumbar spinal stenosis is the most common form of the condition.

Causes of Spinal Stenosis

As people age and lead a unhealthy lifestyle, their spinal discs, which separate the vertebrae, often become less spongy. This can cause them to decrease in size, harden, and bulge into the spinal canal. This can also lead to the formation of spurs, or bony growths, that are harmful to the joints in the spine. In addition chronic stress in the lower back can result in the spinal ligaments becoming thicker and harder. Furthermore, joint disease, or osteoarthritis, can destroy important cushioning in the vertebral column. Finally, arthritic conditions can also cause the bones to thicken. The combination of these factors produces a narrowing of the spinal canal, and this narrowing places pressure on the nerves as they exit the spinal column.

Although younger individuals with developmental problems may suffer from lumbar spinal stenosis, the condition most commonly affects individuals over 60 years of age. Estimates show that as many as 400,000 Americans show signs of lumbar spinal stenosis, and up to 1.2 million Americans suffer from back and leg pain caused by the condition.

Common Symptoms of Spinal Stenosis

While it is not unusual for individuals over the age of 50 to experience some narrowing of the spinal canal, many of them do not show signs symptomatic of lumbar spinal stenosis. When symptoms are present, however, they may include any one or more of the following:

❖ Lower back pain

❖ Leg and thigh stiffness

❖ Numbness, pain, weakness, or cramping in the legs, feet, or buttocks. These sensations may worsen with the extension of the back that occurs when walking standing up straight, or leaning backward, and they may lessen with back flexion, such as occurs when sitting or leaning forward.

❖ Sciatica-like pain radiating into one or both legs

❖ Loss of bladder/bowel control in rare and severe cases

❖ Loss of motor functioning in the legs in rare cases

These symptoms may vary in duration and, when they are present, it is not uncommon for them to vary in severity.

How to Diagnose Spinal Stenosis

Lumbar spinal stenosis can be diagnosed by a chiropractor based on a patient's medical history, a physical examination, and imaging testing including the following:

❖ **X-ray** to examine vertebral and joint structure

❖ **CT scan** to reveal spinal canal shape and size

❖ **MRI** to obtain a three-dimensional image of the spinal cord, including nerve roots, any tumors, and any surrounding abnormalities

❖ **Myleogram**, which is an X-ray of the spinal canal that involves an injection to enable differentiation of areas. A myleogram allows the neurosurgeon to detect pressure on the spinal cord caused by bone spurs, tumors, or herniated discs.

Treatment

Depending on the severity of the condition, treatment options for lumbar spinal stenosis can range from medication or epidural injections to alleviate pain to spine surgery. If back pain is present, the first step in treatment and recovery is accurately diagnosing the cause of the pain. Only then is it possible to determine the best course of action for treating the condition and resuming healthy daily activity.

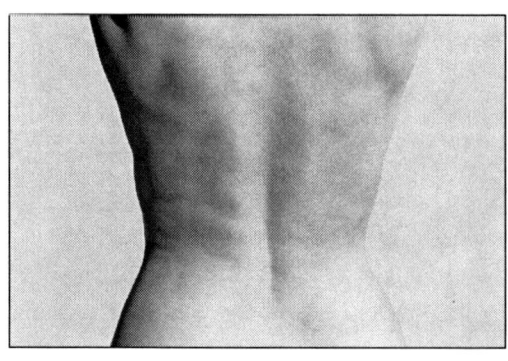

Chronic Back Pain Syndrome: What It Is, What Causes It, and How It Can Be Treated

Chronic back pain is defined as a dull or aching pain in the back that persists for three to six months or longer. Chronic back pain may be contrasted with acute back pain, which usually lasts for only a relatively short period of time ranging from a few days to a few weeks. While nearly every person experiences back pain at some point in his or her life, the pain becomes chronic in less than 10% of these cases.

Although back pain develops into chronic back pain in only a small percentage of the affected population, statistics show that chronic back pain is a major medical concern among individuals in today. According to the Canadian-based Chronic Back Pain Clinic, in North America alone, chronic back pain is among the top five reasons that individuals seek medical care, and as many as 80% of people will visit a doctor at some point in their lives as a result of chronic back pain.

Second Most Common Cause of Missed Work Days

Moreover, chronic back pain is the second most common cause of missed work days, with only the common cold ranking higher. Among money spent on medical care, chronic back pain comes in sixth in total dollars invested, and this painful condition is the third most common reason individuals undergo surgery.

Not a respecter of persons, chronic back pain impacts women and men of all races, and rather than showing indication of improvement, chronic back pain disability rates are worsening at a rate 14 times greater than population growth. It is estimated today that as many as 70 million people in the United States — or as much as 15-30 percent of the US population — suffers from chronic pain. In fact, more people are affected by chronic pain than heart disease or cancer.

These sobering statistics indicate that now more than ever it is vital that we understand this debilitating disease, its causes, and the best mechanisms for treating it.

When Does Your Back Pain Become Chronic?

Back pain can be caused by a variety of factors, including injury, trauma, bone disease, or spinal degeneration occurring over time. When the pain recurs more than three times within a year, or when it lasts longer than three to six months and interferes with regular activities such as sleeping, walking, bending, driving a car, sitting, or standing, it may be classified as chronic.

Chronic pain can be broken down into two categories: pain the source of which is specific (as in an injury) and pain the source of which is not identifiable (such as an injury that has healed). While both conditions technically describe chronic pain, usually the term chronic is used to refer to the latter condition in which the injured tissue has healed, yet the pain persists.

Factors Contributing to Chronic Back Pain

When real pain is present, pain signals are sent to the brain through the nervous system. In some cases, even after the original source of pain is no longer causing pain, the signals continue to be sent. In essence, the pain becomes the condition itself rather than merely a symptom of another condition. Naturally, this prolongs the "chronic" nature of the pain.

Additional physical and psychological factors can also contribute to chronic back pain. For example, physical deconditioning due to lack of exercise plays a key role in causing and prolonging chronic back pain. Exercise, and specifically exercises aimed at strengthening the lower back, can help prevent the onset of back pain and, where pain is present, exercise can help reduce its effects. Conversely, lack of physical exercise can contribute to the continuance of chronic back pain.

Stress Can Cause Chronic Back Pain

Psychologically, mental health can play a key role in causing chronic back pain. In instances in which injury is not present, emotional or mental stress and anxiety can actually bring about chronic back pain. And where pain is already present, an individual's thoughts about the pain, as well as his or her falling into a state of depression and/or anxiety resulting from the pain or other factors, may contribute to prolonged suffering. Researchers estimate that as many as 20 to 50% of individuals with chronic pain also show signs of depression and anxiety.

Best Method to Ending Chronic Back Pain

Because the causes of chronic back pain may extend beyond apparent medical conditions to include emotional and psychological factors, treatment must also go beyond the physical. In addition to prescribed medications to help alleviate pain, a doctor may recommend psychological evaluation and treatment and emotional therapy and support to address the root causes of the pain. In reality, this multidisciplinary approach is the best method in many cases for effectively treating chronic back pain.

In summary, regardless of the initial cause, back pain can become chronic for any number of reasons, including physical, emotional, and psychological in nature. With accurate diagnosis and treatment by an experienced healthcare professional, most cases of chronic back pain can be managed and the ability to live an active and full life restored.

Seven Other Possible Causes of Back Pain

When your chiropractor or doctor evaluates your back pain, you may be required to undergo an initial consultation, a physical examination, and specific tests to help diagnose your condition. There are a number of other possible back conditions that can be contributing to or causing your pain.

Fibromyalgia

A chronic disorder characterized by widespread musculoskeletal pain, fatigue, sleep problems, and morning stiffness, fibromyalgia occurs more often in women between the ages of 20 to 40. The symptoms can be relatively mild in some but severe and disabling in others.

The condition is difficult to diagnose because its symptoms can mimic many other ailments but is generally suspected when a patient has experienced the widespread pain for more than three months. Also characteristic of this disorder is pain when slight pressure is applied to a series of 18 "tender points" found in various locations of the body such as the neck, spine, shoulders and hips. It is generally considered fibromyalgia when 11 of the 18 "tender points" are painful when touched.

The cause of fibromyalgia remains unknown although many researchers suspect a previous injury or trauma, virus, infection, or changes in the autonomic nervous system may be involved. Others believe that fibromyalgia suffers may have a lower threshold for pain due to unusual sensitivity in the brain.

Treatment for fibromyalgia consists of a number of methods aimed at controlling the symptoms since it remains a chronic condition. Some of these are medication, exercise, massage, cognitive behavioral therapy, acupuncture, massage, and chiropractic care.

Transitional Vertebrae

Patients with transitional vertebrae are born with this condition. In the spinal column, there are various types of vertebrae where the ones in the lower back are called "lumbar", the "sacral" are below them.

In transitional vertebrae, one of the vertebra does not form as lumbar or sacral, rather a combination of the two. Thus it has characteristics of both kinds of vertebrae.

Treatment consists of physical therapy to make the back more stable and to increase strength and stability. Braces may also be used to give the back support. Sometimes steroid injections are given to reduce the pain and discomfort that this condition may cause.

Osteomyelitis

Osteomyelitis is an acute chronic inflammatory infection of the bone caused by bacteria. In adults it usually occurs in the vertebrae or pelvis, while in children it is seen in the long bones of the arms and legs.

Patients with osteomyelitis often present with severe pain in the affected bone and the skin directly above the area may be red or swollen. There may also be fever, chills, or nausea.

The infection may develop after an injury or trauma when the bacteria enter the bone through the bloodstream from the wound site. It may also enter the bloodstream from an infection in another area of the body and move into the bone. Some doctors suspect osteomyelitis is caused by the Staphylococcus bacteria.

The condition is diagnosed with blood work to check for infection, bone scans, X-rays, and/or MRI.

Treatment consists of IV antibiotics followed by oral antibiotics. In some rare cases, the infection may require surgery to remove pus, infection, and damaged tissue from the affected area.

Discitis

This is a relatively uncommon condition that can occur in adults, but more often in children under the age of 10. It is an inflammatory infection that affects the disc space between vertebrae. Symptoms usually include slow onset of severe back pain that becomes worse from movement. There may also be symptoms of infection such as fever, chills, sweating, or fatigue.

A diagnosis of discitis is made after imaging tests such as radiograph or MRI where there is evidence of extension of the spine showing disc space narrowing between the vertebrae. Discitis often affects the lumbar (lower) and thoracic (upper) back vertebrae.

Possible causes of discitis are Staphylococcus, viruses, or other inflammatory processes that may create the symptoms.

This condition is treated by immobilizing the back, sometimes with the use of a plaster cast or a specially designed back brace. Some doctors will also prescribe antibiotics to treat the infection and advise the patient to get plenty of rest until the condition is successfully treated and recovery is noted.

Osteoporosis

Affecting more women in later age than men, osteoporosis is becoming a more common condition as the population ages. Osteoporosis causes loss of bone density, which makes the bones much weaker and brittle. Over time, the bones become more prone to fractures and breakage.

There are no obvious signs to alert the patient until an injury draws attention to the condition. As the bones are affected, they become very spongy. In the spine, the vertebrae may collapse causing fractures. The pain radiates from the back to the side and repeated fractures can cause chronic low back pain.

Osteoporosis is diagnosed using X-rays and bone density testing. The goal of treatment is prevention since bone that has been severely weakened over time is very difficult, sometimes impossible to treat. Patients are advised to incorporate a healthy lifestyle including plenty of exercise and good diet. Smoking and excessive use of alcohol is discouraged.

Spina Bifida Occulta

This is a hereditary spinal malformation and birth defect where there is an incomplete closure of the spinal cord and the bones of the spine over the spinal cord are not formed completely.

In spina bifida occulta, there is no opening in the back but the outer part of some of the vertebrae is not completely closed. This is one of the mildest forms of spina bifida and the spinal cord does not protrude through the vertebrae.

The skin above the affected area may look normal or it may have excessive hair growing from it. Dimples or a birthmark may be present as well.

There is no single cause attributed to spina bifida occulta but it is much more common than once thought. Most people with it have no symptoms and a small percentage have serious complications. It is diagnosed with X-rays and MRI where the abnormality can be easily observed. Folic acid has been shown to aid in prevention of the condition and pregnant women are encouraged to add it to their prenatal regimen.

The condition is treated with surgery in serious cases where any opening in the back is closed and medication may be prescribed for those suffering from pain.

Scoliosis

Scoliosis is the most common deformity of the spine. It is generally noticed around adolescence and is an abnormal curvature of the spine. Cases where the curvature is more predominant are found more in girls than boys.

It is diagnosed using X-rays or other imaging techniques but can be readily detected just by observation. There is lateral curvature where the vertebral column appears to bend from side to side and may resemble the letter "S" or "C" when the patient is asked to bend forward. Rotation or a twisting abnormality of the vertebrae is a common observation.

In most cases of scoliosis, the cause is unknown while a smaller number can be associated with abnormal development of the spinal vertebrae or problems in other areas of the body, such as uneven leg length, that affect the curvature of the spine. Patients with severe cases may suffer from back pain and difficulty breathing.

Scoliosis is treated with surgery in some cases to fuse vertebrae into position, as well as braces, chiropractic manipulation and physical therapy. The goal is to diagnose this condition as early as possible since curvature is difficult to correct after the condition has progressed.

Overall ...

Back pain is one of the most common ailments that affect almost everyone at some point in life. While some experience rather mild or short-term suffering, others deal with back pain that becomes chronic and even disabling. A visit to your chiropractor may be a step in the right direction to learn exactly what is going on and how to get relief from back pain.

Important Self-Treatment
Tips for Back Pain

I f you experience back pain from muscle strain or even from a sedentary lifestyle, there is a good chance that relief can be found in your very own home. In fact, there are several effective pain relievers that do not require a prescription. There are also effective stretches and exercises you can do to strengthen your back and decrease pain. They are available at any local drug store, pharmacy, or convenience store. Thus, there are some very basic steps to treating back pain in the comfort of your home.

Even the most cautious people can make a mistake from time to time. If you experience back pain, there are treatment options you can exercise from home. Moreover, not all back pain requires drastic medical intervention. In fact, your body has the capacity to heal itself; many patients find that the pain subsides on its own after a short period of time. However, when the pain is severe and interferes with normal activity, some action must be taken to alleviate it.

Heat and Ice

To start with, heat can be applied with a regular hot water bottle or heating pad. When applied to muscles in the irritated area, heat causes nearby blood vessels to dilate. This helps flush out the vessels and remove chemical irritants that trigger the pain. Meanwhile, ice is as close as your freezer. Of course you also have the option of purchasing ice packs from your local drug store or pharmacy.

At any rate, ice has the opposite effect of heat, causing constriction of the blood vessels. Thus, smaller vessels translate to relief of inflammation and muscle spasms.

While some patients report more pain relief from one of the two treatments, physicians often recommend alternating heat and ice.

The decontamination properties of heat and the anti-inflammatory reaction to cold work well together to reduce pain, particularly during the first few days. Furthermore, there are several different products available that are designed for heat therapy at home.

For example, many patients choose an electric heating pad. The most basic of these devices has low and high settings in addition to the fact that they stay warm until the device is switched off. However, electric heating pads can quickly become fire hazards when they are cracked (often from being folded for storage) or when the electrical cord becomes frayed. They may also ignite a fire when used near machines that store or release oxygen, which is why hospitals avoid them.

Nonetheless, the safest heat therapy tools are those which do not rely on electricity. For instance, microwavable water heating pads or wheat heating pads are very effective. Most importantly, they are not fire hazards and there is very little, if any, risk of thermal burning when microwavable products are used as directed.

Over-the-Counter Pain Relievers

There are a variety of pain relievers available over the counter anywhere from the pharmacy to the convenience store. Though they achieve the same results, it is important to remember that pain relievers are not all alike. For instance, aspirin works primarily as a blood thinner, while other pain relievers are anti-inflammatory drugs with blood-thinning properties.

Some examples of anti-inflammatory drugs include ibuprofen and naproxen. Also, there is a newer type of anti-inflammatory medication known as COX-2 Inhibitors. Brand names of these drugs include Celebrex and Vioxx. Of course, these anti-inflammatory drugs are often preferred over aspirin because they do not have as high a prevalence of gastrointestinal side effects. Still, it is important to note that Vioxx was voluntarily removed from the market by its manufacturer because it has been shown to cause cardiovascular complications.

Though Celebrex is still available, the FDA has requested further research about anti-inflammatory medications. Meanwhile, acetaminophen, known most commonly by the brand name Tylenol, deactivates the brain's perception of pain. Depending on what is best for your health, you may be better served relying not on these types of medications, but finding the cause of your back pain and then fix the underlying problem.

Personal Exercise Program

One of the best ways to relieve chronic back pain is to condition your back muscles.

This means making them more flexible, stronger, and well-conditioned. Fortunately, this does not require you to become a marathon runner. In fact, quite the opposite is necessary for patients with back pain. All that is necessary is an exercise that is paced and appropriate for your current condition. For optimal spinal health, exercises should focus on moderate stretching exercises, core strengthening exercises, and low-impact aerobics. Thus, stretching promotes flexibility, core strengthening helps to stabilize the spinal column, and aerobic training keeps excess weight at a minimum. With a stronger, healthier set of back and abdominal muscles, your chance of experiencing a muscle injury is significantly reduced. This is, of course, due to the fact that strong muscles do not become fatigued and strained as easily. A balanced spine distributes weight evenly throughout the muscles.

Ask Your Doctor

Though home remedies are easy to use and effective, you should always discuss your back pain and possible treatment options with a physician. More than likely, he or she will recommend conservative methods that address your injury, overall health, and lifestyle. In particular, you should always ask a physician when taking medication. He or she has the ability to make the best recommendation based on your medical history, which is essential because of the possible side effects medications may have.

Why Bed Rest Is Bad for Back Pain

For most people, the onset of back pain makes the idea of moving around seem very unappealing. Nevertheless, the first instinct is to rest the muscles and move as little as possible. While this may be a good idea for the first couple of days after a muscle injury, prolonged period of rest can lead to further complications. Most importantly, too much rest often translates to more back pain that ends up lingering longer than it would have if the muscles remained active. This is true because rendering any muscle inactive for an extended period of time causes a loss of flexibility, muscle atrophy, blood clots, and even depression.

Muscle Weakness

The reason bed rest is often so ineffective in treating back pain can be summed up in one sentence: Movement is life. The human body is made for movement. Accordingly, movement keeps the muscles flexible and well-conditioned. In fact, some back pain is actually caused by sedentary living. For example, people who sit for long periods of time during the day have weaker muscles, making them more prone to injury than someone with strong, healthy muscles. Furthermore, there are two basic components of healthy muscles, flexibility, and conditioning.

To begin with, tight, constricted muscles lead to unhealthy imbalances of the spine. When rigid muscles restrict motion, spinal movements become imbalanced, which causes even more back pain. It can cause injuries to surrounding muscles, which may be forced to compensate for the already injured muscles' lack of flexibility. Fortunately, stretching exercises prevent the loss of flexibility, injury to nearby muscles, and any re-injury to the muscle causing the initial pain.

In addition to flexibility, well-conditioned muscles are important to relieving and preventing back pain. As mentioned, weak muscles are more prone to injury in the first place. Prolonged periods of rest will only make the muscle weaker; even if it heals, the likelihood of recurring back pain increases significantly.

Some conditioning exercises can help alleviate back pain sooner. This is due to the fact that conditioning exercises usually entail some light to moderate aerobic activity, which increases circulation. Thus, increased circulation translates to more oxygen for the muscles, which naturally provides pain relief. Also, good circulation will help you avoid painful blood clots, which are typically found in the legs of a patient who has been immobile for an extended period of time. Though blood clots often go unnoticed, they can lead to heart complications in some patients.

Conditioning exercise also strengthens the muscles, which improves spinal stability. Increased stability helps to prevent imbalances of the spine, thus preventing recurring injury. Of course, before attempting any exercise, it is essential that you consult a physician. He or she can assign exercises appropriate for your condition.

The Link Between Back Pain and Depression

Most people are aware that depression can lead to back and neck pain. The mind is powerful when it comes to physical health. In fact, patients who harbor anxiety in their subconscious often experience oxygen deprivation in the muscles. Friends and loved ones around them may be inclined to think of these patients as hypochondriacs, but the pain they experience is real.

The exception is that back pain requires treatment that targets not only the point of injury but also the mental anxiety causing it. Back pain can trigger depression, particularly in patients who are inactive for an extended period of time. Though a few injuries or conditions require prolonged rest periods, it is usually best to resume normal activities as soon as possible.

After all, it is difficult and even depressing to forego hobbies and activities you ordinarily enjoy, especially if it means staying in bed and thinking constantly about the pain you are feeling.

After the Brief Rest Period

Thus, the best solution for back pain is to rest only for a couple of days, possibly relying on conservative therapies such as chiropractic adjustments, core stability exercises, stretches, and heat-ice therapy to alleviate inflammation and flush out toxins. After that, you should do your very best to resume normal activity over the next month or so.

If such activities are still painful, continue to make use of conservative treatments that ease your pain. For example, if your hobby is gardening, you should consider wearing a back brace to provide more support and stability for your spine. You may also find relief from medications until the muscles regain their flexibility and strength. Of course, it is also important not to overdo activities that are hard on your back, especially too soon after the injury. One way to address this concern is to decrease the amount of time you spend in the garden each day.

However, if your physician recommends that you discontinue a particular set of activities for an extended period of time, you can still resume normal daily activities. Most importantly, you will be better served just to leave your home and be around positive things that take your mind off the pain. Interpersonal communication, for instance, can be very therapeutic.

Chances are, friends, and family will help encourage you to get out of bed so they may enjoy your company. And it is highly unlikely they will be eager to discuss your back pain, which means you will not have to dwell on it unnecessarily as you would if staying at home in bed.

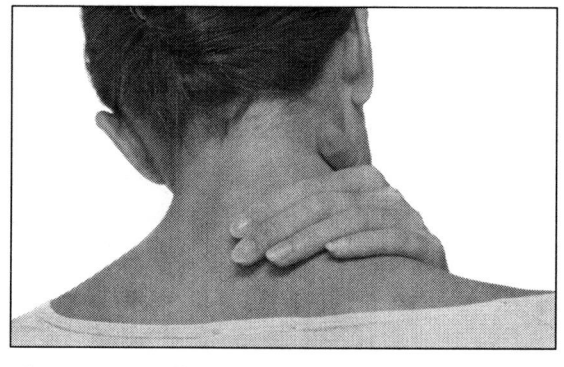

From Cervical to Lumbar: The Spine Is Affected by Your Slumber

During sleep, you are very likely to remain in the same position for several hours at a time. So if you are sleeping in the wrong position, your spine becomes imbalanced. This causes stiff, strained muscles and potentially severe pain the next morning.

Many patients with back pain are completely unaware that their sleep positions are either causing or worsening their discomfort. In fact, changing the position in which you sleep may be all it takes to alleviate back pain for good. This may seem too good to be true. But the simple precautions you take can often have a major and long-lasting impact on your health.

For example, you may be personally aware that back pain causes sleep deprivation. However, are you also aware that sleep deprivation may lead to obesity? And obesity can cause back pain because the extra weight places excessive pressure on the spine. There are a few simple changes that anyone can make to keep the spine in a neutral position during the night. These changes are subtle, yet they make a tremendous difference for you.

First and foremost, it is crucial that the spine remains in an "S" shape. Fortunately, a very healthy position for slumber is on your side, which is also known as the fetal position. In order to achieve this, simply lie on your side with a pillow under your head (for neck support) and a pillow between your knees, which should be slightly drawn toward your chest.

Thus, many patients compare this to a fetal position. There are many retailers that offer pillows designed for a patient to "hug," placing them between the knees and holding onto them with their arms. Though they are commonly used by pregnant women, they are useful for anyone with back pain. This position is very effective in relieving back pain for patients suffering from spinal stenosis, osteoarthritis of the spine, or hip pain.

The Best Sleeping Posture Even If You Are Pregnant

Physicians also suggest that pregnant women sleep on the side, particularly the left side. This is due to the fact that the major blood vessels are located on the right side; therefore, lying on the left side reduces pressure on these vessels and allows for maximum blood flow and circulation.

Not only is this beneficial for the fetus, good circulation is beneficial for the woman and the muscles throughout her body (more oxygen means less pain). Furthermore, back sleeping leads to unnecessary pressure on the inferior vena cava, a major vessel that delivers blood from the lower part of her body to the heart.

Still, not everyone is comfortable lying on the side. Fortunately, physicians have recommendations for such patients. For instance, if you elect to slumber while lying on your back, just place a pillow beneath your knees in addition to a small pillow under your lower back. This position can be very effective in alleviating lower back discomfort.

The Sleeping Position You Should Avoid at All Cost ...

Sleeping on your belly is not recommended due to the fact that it forces you to turn your head sideways. You may even twist your back slightly without even realizing it. Nevertheless, this twisting is unnatural and unhealthy for your spine.

If you must rest on your abdomen, there is one way to make it much easier on the spine. If you choose to sleep face down, just place a pillow beneath your pelvis and lower abdomen. If you sleep with a pillow beneath your head, make sure it is not creating unnecessary strain on your back. If your suspect it may be causing a strain, try sleeping without it. Instead, sleep only with a pillow placed beneath the pelvis.

What You Should Know About Your Mattress

If you find that changing the sleeping position does not provide relief for your back pain, the source of your discomfort may be your mattress. Though many manufacturers advertise mattresses designed to support the spine and improve sleep quality, no one mattress is recommended for all patients with back pain. Instead, most patients find that the proper mattress is actually a question of personal preference.

Still, many patients with chronic back pain find relief when they try a medium-firm mattress. If you would like to experience a firmer mattress without purchasing one or waiting for a trial offer, simply place a piece of plywood beneath the mattress. If you find that the back pain is reduced, keep the plywood there until you decide to purchase a firmer mattress.

An adjustable bed may also be a good investment. This is true because an adjustable bed can help neutralize the spine for patients who prefer to lie on their backs. With this type of bed, there would no longer be a need for strategically placed pillows.

Though sleeping positions may seem like a minor detail, proper positioning is very essential to maintaining a healthy spine as well as good overall health. It is important to remember that most people do not move very often during sleep.

If you are in a position that compromises spinal balance, you will probably be there for a long time. During that time, your muscles will remain in an unnatural position, become strained, stiffened, and cause you pain the next day. Moreover, once the back pain has begun, you may find it difficult to sleep at all, which can negatively affect your overall wellbeing.

How to Get Out of Bed the *Right* Way

One of the most successful means of treating back pain is preventing it from occurring in the first place. Fortunately, this does not mean restricting your activity. Instead, it can simply mean going about your daily activities in a different way.

Simple details such as how you stand, sit, and get out of bed each day can dramatically reduce the amount of back pain you experience. Just as are there simple ways to alleviate back pain, there are also very fundamental steps you can take to prevent back pain from occurring or recurring.

To avoid back pain you should learn the basic techniques or ergonomics of the human body in relation to preventing muscle strain, particularly on the back. Following are a few examples of preventative measures you can take.

The Best Way to Get Up from a Lying/Prone Position

When you wake up in the morning or rise from an afternoon nap, you do not really think about how you will get out of bed. If you are suffering from back pain you may even dread the idea of getting out of bed knowing that it will be very uncomfortable, since lying down for an extended period of time causes the muscles to become stiff.

However, there are a few undemanding steps you can take to make getting up much easier. To begin with, lie on your side facing the side of the bed where you plan to get out. This helps to prevent unnecessary twisting of the back and pelvis.

Next, lower your legs to the floor, making sure you do not fall. It is essential that you keep your back straight. And finally, use the arm beneath you to gradually push your body upward. When this endeavor is completed, you should be in a sitting position.

Give Your Back Muscles a Rest While Standing

Perhaps you work in the retail industry and must stand for long periods of time each day. Or maybe you work in the food industry with a supervisor and a "no sitting policy."

Whatever the occupation, this can be hard on the lower back muscles. Still, there is one simple way for you to provide relief. Simply rest one leg on a footstool, alternating feet throughout the day.

Let Your Back Muscles Take a Rest While Sitting

Though you may be inclined to assume that sitting automatically means relief, sitting incorrectly can cause pain just as easily as standing improperly. People with desk jobs must pay special attention to how they sit each day. Fortunately, there are a few straightforward ways to ease the strain on back muscles while sitting.

First, it is essential to choose a supportive chair, especially if you must remain in it for long periods of time. A good chair must have good lower back support, arm rests and a base that swivels.

Additionally, it is important to help the spine maintain its normal curve. You can achieve this by placing a rolled towel or pillow at the small of the back. Lastly, remember to keep your knees and hips level.

For instance, do not be tempted to rest your feet on that troublesome box of copy paper sitting below your desk. This will bring your knees too high. In fact, it is always best to keep such objects out from under the desk in the first place. People sitting in chairs too high for them find that their knees are too far below their hips.

What You Should Know About Lifting

Improper lifting is a common cause of back pain among all types of patients. One of the most important steps any patient can take is to make sure not to lift an object that is too heavy. When in doubt, swallow your pride and ask for help.

If you decide you are able to lift the object, remember these basic techniques:

1. To begin with, the closer you can get your body to whatever it must lift, the better off your muscles. In order to truly avoid back pain, practice this technique with everything you lift, whether it is a basket of laundry or a heavy piece of furniture.

2. In addition, be sure to lift with your legs rather than your back, which is best accomplished by lifting in a vertical motion.

3. It is crucial that you avoid twisting you body as you lift. If you must turn, lift the object and then move your feet, keeping your spine properly aligned.

It Is Never Too Late

Even if you have been challenged in more than one of these areas, you will be better served by taking these precautions in your everyday lifestyle. They are all perfect examples of how the small details can make a significant difference in your health. Most importantly, whether you are young or old, it is never too late or too early to learn the proper mechanics when it comes to rising, standing, sitting, and lifting.

Hot or Cold? How This Household Remedy Can Alleviate Back Pain

Among the many different conservative treatments, heat and ice therapies are effective for several reasons. First of all, heat therapy helps the body cleanse irritated muscles by dilating blood vessels. As the harmful toxins are removed, pain is eased.

Ice therapy causes the vessels to narrow, which reduces inflammation and muscle spasms. Moreover, this is an effective treatment option because it is non-invasive and safe for nearly all patients. For example, unlike medications, there is no risk for side effects when used properly.

This means that patients who are taking medications for other health issues can find pain relief without worrying about how the treatment will interact with other drugs. Still, heat and ice is often prescribed in combination with medication as well as other treatments.

Heat and ice are also successful in relieving back pain when they are used together. In fact, many physicians encourage patients to alternate between these two therapies for optimal results. Of course, before using heat and ice together, it is best to have a thorough understanding of how they work individually.

When You Should Use Only Ice

First and foremost, it is essential that only ice is used to treat acute back pain during the initial 48-hour period following the injury. Ice is most effective for acute pain due to muscle strain or spasms because of its anti-inflammatory properties. For example, if you can feel that you have pulled a muscle, one of the first things you can do is use an ice pack on the sore area.

A home-made ice pack right from your freezer will do the trick but there are also gel packs available at local drug stores. Applying heat too soon may add to existing inflammation because it triggers dilation of the vessels. Therefore, wait 48 hours before applying any heat to the area.

When You Should Start Using Heat

Once 48 hours have passed, you may want to introduce heat to the sore muscles. Most patients find that alternating ice and heat provide effective pain relief. To do this, simply apply ice for 20 minutes and then heat for 20 minutes.

Then, you should repeat this process every two hours. Accordingly, the ice will shrink the blood vessels and reduce swelling, and the heat will enlarge the vessels and flush out the harmful chemicals that have built up in your muscles as a result of the injury. Of course, heating pads can be found at local drugs stores and they are fairly easy to use. However, when using a heating pad, there are important precautions you must take.

Read This Before You Start Using Heat

First, it is crucial that you inspect the heating pad before each use. If it appears cracked or otherwise worn out, do not use it. You should also check the electric cord for any signs of fraying.

While it may seem overly cautious to check the device each time, it is important because heating pads can easily start a fire. In fact, people have been seriously and even fatally injured in fires caused by heating pads, according to the FDA. Many of these individuals were over the age of 65 and/or hospitalized; thus, if you are a caretaker for an elderly person, remember to check the heating pad before allowing them to use it.

Caretakers should also remember not to use this device near equipment which stores or releases oxygen. It is also important to properly maintain your heating pad. For example, do not fold the heating pad or bend it for any reason. This prevents cracking that can lead to a fire.

If you decide to use a heating pad that may be old, take a moment to consider whether it will be safer to replace the device with a newer one. Purchasing a new heating pad may be a much safer choice than using an older one which may have deteriorated if it has been stored away for a long period of time.

Nevertheless, most heating pad burns do not occur with fire but from the instrument itself. This is because many people use heating pads at night. This can lead to problems for several reasons.

1. To begin with, you should never lie on a heating pad. For example, if you are using the device to apply heat to the lower back, lie on your side and drape the heating pad over the sore muscles.

2. You may get better results if you lie on your abdomen and allow the heating pad to rest on your lower back. Of course, abdomen sleeping is very hard on the lower back. If you must sleep this way in order to use the heating pad, remember to place a pillow below your pelvis. Still, it is best not sleep in this position for an extended period of time.

3. Most importantly, remember that thermal burns can occur even when a heating pad is turned to the lowest setting. Many people use these devices overnight, thinking that they are safe from burns if they keep the heat at the lowest setting.

4. The use of sleep aids increases the chances of being injured by a heating pad. This situation certainly applies to patients with back pain because many of them take sleep medication. Otherwise, their pain may keep them from getting any rest. The FDA does not recommend the use of heating pads by patients on sleep medication.

5. Also, people with skin desensitized from spinal cord injuries or diabetes, as well as elderly persons, are at particular risk of getting a thermal burn from one of these devices. In fact, the FDA advises these patients to avoid heating pads entirely.

Still, there are other options for patients who may benefit from heat therapy. In fact, microwavable heating pads and hot water bottles work well for everyone, especially patients who experience limited feeling in the skin.

The Good, The Bad, and The Ugly of Anti-Inflammatory Drugs

Anti-inflammatory drugs are commonly prescribed for patients suffering from back pain. This is true because injuries cause the muscles to become inflamed, causing the area to become tight and irritated. The patients lose flexibility and often find the most basic everyday activities are difficult.

Furthermore, many physicians recommend that anti-inflammatory drugs be taken along with pain relievers such as acetaminophen because they are effective in reducing swelling while other pain relievers work more like numbing agents. For example, acetaminophen works in the brain, deactivating it from pain sensations caused by nerve pressure.

Since it does not reduce the swelling that causes nerve pressure, doctors typically recommend that patients alternate or take anti-inflammatory medications with pain relievers like acetaminophen.

Both types of medication are available over the counter and by prescription, depending on the strength necessary to treat the injured muscle. Still, you should consult your physician not only to determine whether these medications are right for you but also to consider other treatment options.

Do You Want to Fix or Patch Your Back Pain?

While anti-inflammatory medications are effective for many patients, they do not always address the source of your back pain. In some cases, injuries are incidental and medications provide pain relief while the body works to promote self-healing.

However, in other cases, drugs only neutralize the pain without addressing its source.

For example, if you suffer from chronic or recurring back pain, you should consider incorporating an exercise routine into your daily lifestyle. After all, exercise helps to increase flexibility in addition to strengthening, stabilizing, and conditioning the muscles. Thus, the muscles are less likely to become strained and create imbalances in the spine.

Back pain may also be triggered by vertebral subluxation, which is simply blockages that disrupt healthy communication within the nervous system. The best way to address these subluxations is to seek chiropractic care. This is true because chiropractors specialize in relieving pain caused by subluxations in order to allow the body to heal itself.

Whatever the case may be, it is always best to locate and treat the source of back pain rather than just dulling it temporarily. It may take time and a little more work on your part; nevertheless, you are far more likely to experience permanent pain relief. And possibly end the battle with back pain.

Medications alleviate pain, particularly during its acute phase, but the discomfort will only return when the weakened muscle becomes strained and irritated again. Anti-inflammatory drugs are not effective when taken as needed for pain relief. Instead, patients are advised to take them regularly so that the prescribed dosage can built up within the body over a period of time.

So you are faced with a question of whether to manage pain by masking it or by treating its cause. Of course, there are side effects that every patient should consider before taking anti-inflammatory medication.

Potential Side Effects of Anti-Inflammatory Medication

In order to understand the potential risk factors involved with taking medication, it is important to recognize that there are different types of anti-inflammatory drugs available. First of all, NSAIDs (non-steroidal anti-inflammatory drugs) are among those most commonly prescribed. These include ibuprofen and naproxen. They work like aspirin but usually have a lower risk of gastrointestinal side effects.

Aspirin is a blood thinner, which means it can damage the lining of a patient's stomach and lead to peptic ulcers. Additionally, COX-2 Inhibitors are a new group of NSAIDs. They work by preventing the chemical reaction that causes inflammation rather than working to stop the formation of inflammation like traditional NSAIDs.

Also, COX-2 Inhibitors do not hamper the production of stomach lining; thus, they are associated with fewer cases of stomach ulcers. Still, both NSAIDs and COX-2 Inhibitors carry a risk of side effects of which every patient should be aware before taking them.

To begin with, ibuprofen and naproxen (both are NSAIDs) have blood-thinning properties and are not recommended for patients with sensitive stomachs or existing ulcers. Even if you have a healthy stomach, you will be better served if you take NSAIDs with food. This helps to ease any irritation to your gastrointestinal system. NSAIDs should also be avoided by people who take other blood thinning drugs because unnecessary blood thinning can trigger bleeding.

Ibuprofen can diminish the effectiveness of diuretics and some blood pressure medications. Meanwhile, naproxen can lead to potentially fatal interaction when taken with MAOIs (monoamine oxidase inhibitors) like Marplan and Nardil.

COX-2 Inhibitors have another slate of potential side effects. Most notably, they have been shown to cause cardiovascular problems in some patients. The popular drug known as Vioxx was voluntarily removed from the market by its manufacturer.

Long-term usage of this type of medication has also been shown to cause problems with the gastrointestinal system along with the liver and kidneys. These complications are particularly evident among elderly patients due to the fact that COX-2 Inhibitors are commonly prescribed for arthritis. In order to determine whether you are at risk for these side effects, it is best to speak with your physician.

In truth, your physician or specialist is the best person to help you determine whether an anti-inflammatory in any form is best for you. For example, he or she may recommend that you take an anti-inflammatory for a short period of time as you begin your new exercise routine. This would help alleviate the initial inflammation and pain as your body becomes strong and well-conditioned.

Slow and Steady Wins
The Race Against Back Pain

When dealing with a flare up of back pain, whether it is for the first time or one of several occasions, patients are told that they need to become active after only a couple of days rest. This may be difficult to imagine and most people are uncertain about how much activity they should participate in.

Fortunately, there are some straightforward approaches that you can take as you work toward recovering and regaining your active lifestyle. You will find that most, if not all, physicians advocate a slow but steady approach to recovering from back pain. This helps to heal the damaged area completely and without the risk of re-injury.

Start with Small Movements

One of the first steps you can take to transition from bed rest to normal life is to reintroduce small movements. For example, you can start by performing simple, controlled stretching exercises in order to restore flexibility and ease the pain of stiff muscles. These exercises can help the pain to disappear more quickly.

That is why inactive people will experience a longer episode of back pain. It is beneficial to reintroduce regular activities that you are used to performing in your daily lifestyle. For instance, wake up and perform all the necessary tasks of getting dressed without any assistance from another person.

Try to get dressed the way you normally do. As you do this, be sure to listen to your body. If you feel a need to rest for a few minutes in between activities, you should certainly rest. After all, you do not want to risk re-injury to the damaged muscle.

Continue performing small tasks throughout the day but continue to avoid bending and twisting motions. Within a couple of weeks, your daily routine will become natural once again.

Take a Peaceful Walk

Once you are reacquainted with your everyday lifestyle, you may begin adding strengthening and conditioning exercise to your regimen. Walking is among the most beneficial exercises you can perform to alleviate back pain. This is true because walking is a low-impact aerobic activity.

Low impact means just what it says: Unlike jogging and running, walking does not impact the joints. Walking also helps you to slowly regain your range of motion, strengthen core muscles and improve posture. It also strengthens muscles in the legs, hips, abdomen, and back, which stabilizes the spine. Thus, it helps to prevent imbalances that lead to spinal injuries.

Walking enhances circulation, which helps the body to flush out chemical impurities that build up in the muscles as a result of back pain. While there are several other low-impact aerobic activities with these characteristics, walking is favored by many physicians because it is an exercise you can perform anywhere.

For instance, if you have a desk job, you may find sitting in an office building all day leaves your muscles stiff. It is becoming more common to see many office employees use part of their lunch breaks to take walks around or outside the office building.

It is important not to feel shy or embarrassed about adding such a routine to your workday. In fact, unless you work in a small office, most people are not likely to notice what you are doing. In any case, you can make this workout more on the leisurely side and save intensity for the walking track or treadmill.

Is It True What They Say About "No Pain, No Gain"?

While the "no pain, no gain" cliché remains popular among competitive athletes, this approach certainly does not apply to patients recovering from back pain. Aside from the mild soreness you may experience the day or two after your first workout; you should not encounter back pain that is more severe than before the exercise began.

Remember, you are making the effort to treat the back pain, not reignite it. Nevertheless, if the activity only intensifies your pain and inflammation, you should consult your physician. You may have taken on too much too soon and your physician or specialist can redirect you to a more appropriate course of action.

Strengthen Your Core Muscles

As you learn more about the cause of back pain and how to prevent it from becoming chronic or recurring, you need to pay more and more attention to the core stability muscles. These include muscles of the abdomen and back.

Moreover, they are referred to as the core because all movement originates from these 29 important muscles. A strong core ensures that the spine is stabilized and movements are balanced, which prevents re-injury. Core strengthening exercises are non-aerobic.

They include abdominal crunches as well as bridge, plank, and quadruped exercises. The training program known as Pilates is likely to include exercises such as these because it is centered on building a strong core. Yoga classes and workouts with an exercise ball have also become popular form of exercise for improving core strength.

No matter which approach is most appealing, you will be better served to talk with a physician before beginning a core strengthening program and, of course, listen for your body's cues when it comes to the amount of exertion you should apply.

How to Choose a Good Chiropractor

The decision to visit a chiropractor for your back pain may be one of the best choices in your search for relief. A chiropractor can offer you a range of treatment options for your condition and may be able to correct your back pain without surgery or other invasive therapies.

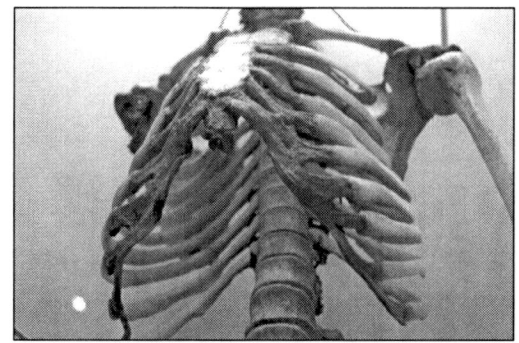

Chiropractic care is becoming one of the most affordable and effective methods for treatment of back pain and related symptoms. During your initial consultation with your chiropractor, he or she will go through a detailed set of questions designed to gain a thorough knowledge of your past and present medical history, as well as any other factors that may be contributing to your condition. This is necessary to determine which chiropractic treatment would be most beneficial for your back pain.

Some Common Questions Your Chiropractor Might Ask

1. Do you have any diagnosed illnesses or conditions?
2. Are you currently taking any medication or other treatments?

One of the most crucial questions is related to your past medical history. This is a very important diagnostic tool because it gives your chiropractor a much better look into how your current back pain may be related to, or caused by, previous health conditions or illnesses. It also provides necessary information for the kind of chiropractic treatment that would be safe and effective based on your current health status.

3. When and how did your back pain start?

Your chiropractor will need to know how and when your back pain started. Treatment for a condition that is of short term or from a known cause may be approached differently than one that has been ongoing for a lengthy period of time or of unknown cause.

A detailed description about the onset of the pain can also be useful as your chiropractor may be able to determine if the condition will be likely to resolve with minimal treatment or if it will require more extensive chiropractic care.

Previous Injury

4. Have you experienced any kind of injury in that past?

5. What treatment did you receive for it?

Sometimes, previous injuries which are considered healed in the past may suddenly resurface as the same area of the back is re-injured or flares up again. There may also be some damage that has left that particular area more susceptible to injury or pain. Other treatment received may also be important as well. Your chiropractor will take all of that into consideration as treatment for your back pain is based in part on your past injuries.

Symptoms

6. What kind of symptoms have you been experiencing?

Often, your chiropractor can assess your condition and the reasons for your back pain depending on the kind of symptoms you are experiencing. Many common back ailments have a group of particular symptoms that the chiropractor will immediately recognize and treat accordingly. Symptoms may also indicate whether your back pain can be effectively treated with chiropractic care or if you may need to seek out other kinds of treatment.

Frequency and Severity of Pain

7. When is your pain worse?

8. How frequent is the pain?

9. Describe it on a scale from zero to ten, ten being worst.

How often and how long the pain lasts can be very good indicators of the source of the problem as well as how to treat it. Many chiropractors use a "pain scale" where the patient is asked to report the degree and frequency of the pain.

For example, they may ask you to judge on a scale from zero to ten, with ten being the worst pain, which level your pain is at, or how often the pain lasts. If it is constant, aching pain, you may say that today it is a "9" or if the pain lasts in short duration, you may say today is an "8" but last week it was only a "3".

Movement

10. Is there any particular movement that initiates or worsens the back pain?

If movement is a factor in your back pain, your chiropractor will need to know if there is any specific kind of movement that initiates or worsens the back pain. This may indicate what kind of condition or injury could be causing your back pain. When movement creates worsening or brings on a bout of pain, there could be certain muscles or bones that are affected and may require a specific chiropractic treatment.

Day-to-day Experience

11. How does the pain affect your everyday life?

12. How do you currently deal with it?

A general summary of how you deal with your back pain on a day-to-day basis can be very useful in developing a treatment plan for you. If you report that your back pain becomes so severe that you end up in bed for days at a time may require different treatment than pain that is only minor and does not affect your daily activity. Ways that you respond to and attempt to control the pain on your own may also give your chiropractor some insight into your experience.

Effect on Mood and Relationships

13. Do you find that your back pain affects your mood or any of your relationships?

If the back pain is having a ripple effect on your ability to function in your everyday life, it must be addressed and taken into account as you explain both your physical and emotional symptoms to your chiropractor. All of the symptoms may be caused by a physical condition or your back pain may be triggering increased stress that affects your mood and relationships.

Since there are so many factors involved in determining the reason(s) and/or kind of condition causing your back pain, the initial consultation with your chiropractor is a very important first step in assessing the best possible chiropractic care needed for your individual situation. Once the chiropractor has all of the necessary information, relief from back pain may be initiated with chiropractic treatment.

Physical Exam: Assessment of Your Back Pain

A thorough physical examination by your chiropractor is one of the most important and necessary means of accurately assessing your condition and possible reasons for your back pain. This is usually completed after your initial consultation and may involve a series of physical tests to help the chiropractor decide which tests or treatment may be most appropriate for you.

While most mainstream medical doctors will generally do a limited physical examination, obtain a brief history of your back pain and, in most cases, write a prescription, a chiropractor will include a much more detailed assessment. It may include a full physical exam, neurological and orthopedic tests, plus specific lab work.

Getting Started: Routine Physical Testing

After an initial interview with your chiropractor in which you explain details of your ailment (how it started, symptoms, what make it worse…), some routine physical testing will generally follow.

This may include checking your weight, blood pressure, temperature, pulse, or basic reflex testing. These are all necessary to give your chiropractor a general idea of basic functioning and may also alert him or her of other conditions that may require a referral to other healthcare practitioners.

If conditions or symptoms that are not within the scope of chiropractic care are suspected, the chiropractor will be very willing to advise you of other kinds of care that may be required. For example, if you have high blood pressure or evidence of a more serious chronic condition, you may need to consult with another healthcare professional.

Full Physical, Neurological and Orthopedic Exam

A series of physical tests will follow and may include specialized physical, neurological, and orthopedic exams in the chiropractor's office. They are generally simple and straightforward but can give the chiropractor a great deal of information about your condition and what is causing the back pain.

Physical Testing

1. **Range of Motion**   You may be asked to perform a series of simple movements so that your chiropractor can observe how effectively you are able to use various parts of your body. For range of motion, you may be asked to bend forward or backward, raise and lower your arms and legs, or tilt your head left or right, forward or backward. You may not need to do all of these movements depending on your particular symptoms and back pain.

2. **Posture**   Poor posture can lead to a variety of back problems and the chiropractor can quickly see if it may be causing some of your back pain. You may be asked to stand normally and then stretch upward or downward, bend forward or backward, or sit then rise. Then report any pain after each test.

Orthopedic / Neurological Testing

3. **Gait Examination**   The patient is asked to walk or march across the room. The chiropractor can observe how smoothly the movement is and if there may be problems in the pelvis or spine.

4. **Palpation of Muscles and Spinal Joints**   Muscles and joints are checked through physical manipulation as the chiropractor places his or her hands on specific locations to check position and condition. Back pain may be caused by muscles and joints in other areas such as the neck, legs or pelvis. Often, a chiropractor can palpate various areas and detect abnormalities such as swelling or bones/joints out of place.

5. **Straight Leg Test**   While the patient is lying down or seated, the doctor raises one leg (at a time) with the knee in a locked position and the hip flexed. If the patient experiences pain, it is suggestive of disc herniation.

6. **Lasegue Test**   The Lasegue Test, also known as Bragard's Test, is conducted with the patient lying down on the back. The leg is flexed and when the knee is extended, there is pain. Or, as the unaffected leg is raised, there may be pain in the other leg. These results are indicative of disc herniation or spinal cord nerve root compression.

7. **Muscle Strength Test**   The patient is asked to raise one leg and the chiropractor will push to create resistance. This provides information on strength, pain, or imbalance in the joints between vertebrae. Muscle testing may also be done in the hands to assess grip strength, sensation, or stiffness that may be associated with a pinched nerve or root compression.

8. **Reflext Test**   Reflex tests are simple physical tests to assess nervous system function. When a joint is tapped with a rubber mallet, the presence or absence of reflex is a good indicator of specific conditions. Response for the deep tendon reflex is a good indicator of nerve damage. A weak or absent response may suggest nerve damage outside the spinal cord while an increased response may indicate spinal cord damage above the level controlling hyperactive response.

9. **Neurological Test for Lower Extremity**   While some of the tests for neurological lower extremity include reflex testing, the patient may also be tested for sensory response, which may indicate damage to the sensory nerves. Most often, the patient will be asked to close his or her eyes and the chiropractor will lightly prick the area with a small steel pin. The presence of pain or absence of feeling may indicate damage to the sciatic nerve or a pinched nerve.

Lab Work

Along with the various physical tests, the chiropractor may also want to order lab tests relevant to your back pain and condition. These can give important information on the three main body systems and determine how efficiently they are working for you. They are your hormonal and immune, digestive, and detoxification systems.

1. **Hormonal and Immune System**   These tests offer information on how imbalances in your hormonal system may be contributing to the physical symptoms that are causing pain and discomfort. Problems in the immune system may create an inability to maintain a strong resistance and balanced bodily functioning. Abnormalities in either of these areas can create havoc in the body.

2. **Digestive System**   The effects of stress and poor eating habits may be seen most often in the digestive system. *Since this system is key to overall body wellness and function,* problems in this area may need to be addressed so that other physical symptoms may be eliminated.

3. **Detoxification System**   Over time, a variety of factors including eating habits and weight, lifestyle, stress, exposure to pollution and toxic chemicals, and even genetics may cause a virtual "build-up" of bad compounds in the body. This can affect any part of the body or system and create a number of symptoms. After detoxification, one is able to function much more efficiently, both mentally and physically.

Completion of Testing

The wide range of physical testing completed by your chiropractor can ensure that any contributing factor or condition relating to your back pain is identified and addressed. There are many individual factors that can be directly or indirectly related to your back pain. Once all of them have been tested, a more specialized, focused treatment plan may be put into motion.

Whole Body Examination: The Mind and Body Connection

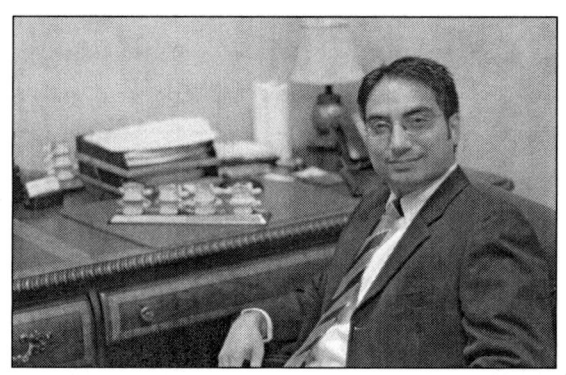

What happens if your chiropractor has done a complete physical examination, lab work, X-rays and MRI but found no physiological reason for your back pain? Since the pain is still present and you are in need of relief, your chiropractor may begin to look for other reasons for your condition.

In spite of the results of your physical testing, there are many other things that may be causing your body to exhibit a variety of symptoms. Chronic or persistent bouts of back pain is one of the most common complaints by patients even when there appears to be no physical evidence to explain why it is occurring.

Psychology of Back Pain

Many patients, who report to chiropractors for treatment of back pain, learn that there is no clear physical reason. But there may be plenty of other factors involved that can explain the pain.

The connection between body and mind is very powerful and your chiropractor may work with you to determine what is really causing your back pain so that you may be able to experience relief. Some of the most common factors contributing or causing back pain are stress and anxiety, emotional issues, mental exhaustion, and negative thinking.

Stress and Anxiety

When a person experiences consistently high levels of stress or anxiety, the body begins to respond with physical symptoms. As the brain becomes "overloaded" with a steady barrage of negative stimuli, it responds by sending excessive adrenalin to various areas of the body.

This is called the "fight or flight" response. When presented with highly stressful stimuli, the brain prepares the body to take action. With continual stress or anxiety, the body begins to become affected and responds with a range of physical symptoms, such as chronic back pain.

Emotional Issues

It has long been known and accepted that significant emotional issues can cause physical symptoms. Take for example how a person who has just experienced a stressful event may become instantly nauseous or faint. Or a person who has a stressful or negative event from his or her past that has not been properly addressed may exhibit many physical symptoms without a medical reason for them. This condition may be diagnosed as "psychosomatic" where there are physical symptoms, but no physical reason for them.

Back pain may be a physical symptom of an underlying emotional issue. Unresolved anger, anxiety, depression or guilt can be presented as pain, and without proper treatment or therapy to control these emotions, the physical symptoms may become chronic and even disabling.

Mental Exhaustion

As each person is unique, so is his or her ability to control and adapt to the ever-changing daily activity in a complex and highly competitive environment. When a person continues to add more and more mental tasks with overwork without proper relief, the result can be mental exhaustion. The body reacts with negative physical symptoms.

Negative Thinking

Many people underestimate the great power of the mind. A pattern of negative thinking can create a negative bodily response. If a person continually thinks that everything will result in a negative outcome or that a minor event will surely become a major tragic event, the mind may make it a self-fulfilling prophecy. Learning to control your thought processes may yield very positive results in many physical symptoms.

Treating Back Pain with No Identifiable Physical Cause

Cognitive Behavioral Therapy

One of the most popular techniques used to help those suffering from physical symptoms where there is no known physical cause is "cognitive behavior therapy." It is a form of psychotherapy based on the assumption that thought can largely determine how we feel. When a patient learns how to control the ways in which the brain processes information and some stimuli, their behavior and overall sense of wellness improves.

If stress and anxiety are reasons for your back pain, cognitive behavioral therapy may be able to help by teaching you better ways of responding to stressors that may help control or prevent the back pain. Changing the ways in which your mind interprets or processes these things can truly help how your body responds to them.

Exercise

If your back pain exists where there is no physical cause, the best treatment may be to add some physical therapy. Many alternative methods of healing are based on the mind-body connection and how achieving balance in both is the key to overall health and wellness. When the mind is not clear and relaxed, neither is the body.

Regular exercise and stretching can be an excellent way to release stress and anxiety while at the same time helping your back pain. The physical movement can strengthen your muscles and increase flexibility.

Your mind may benefit from a new sense of peacefulness as the kind of exercises you choose can be very relaxing and have an overall calming effect. No matter what kind of exercise, it is very useful for both the body and mind.

A Final Note

Even if your back pain has no apparent physical cause, your chiropractor may be able to suggest various other treatment options. Regardless of the real reason for your pain, it exists. Relief can be found in a variety of ways; it is simply a matter of determining which one is right for you.

Final Thoughts on Working with a Chiropractic Doctor

When choosing a chiropractic doctor for your back pain, there are several considerations relevant to your particular situation. Your decision will determine the kind of care you receive and how satisfied you are with the chiropractor. Ultimately, you are placing your trust in his or her professional experience to provide the best possible treatment for your back pain.

The relationship between you and your chiropractor must be positive, beneficial, and professional. The chiropractor and his office staff all play an important role in your ability to achieve health and wellness. After all, it is their business to ensure that all aspects of your chiropractic care meet your expectations and that you are a satisfied patient.

Talking to Your Chiropractor One-on-One

A good chiropractor will give you the necessary information and provide an explanation. An excellent chiropractor will work with you so that you are clear on every detail of your diagnosis and treatment plan. She will be pleased to talk with you and explain everything so that you understand your condition and how the doctor will proceed. She will make you feel comfortable and welcome your questions and concerns.

There should be no pressure or a "rushed" attitude when you are discussing your back pain with your chiropractor. The best chiropractors will feel no need to get through the appointment as quickly as possible. Each patient should be given a reasonable amount of time to ask any questions he may have and receive clear and concise answers.

A knowledgeable chiropractor will want to get a whole, clear picture of your current health status and reason why you have decided to consult his practice. She will be very interested in your case and be ready to conduct appropriate tests or treatments that will be able to address your back pain.

It Is Your Choice

When your chiropractor determines the reason for your back pain, he or she may present more than one treatment option. Top chiropractic doctors involve the patient in which course to follow. They present the choices and are fully prepared to discuss the advantages and disadvantages of each.

Plus, they can give the patient their professional opinion, but it remains the patient's final decision. Rarely is there only one choice, although there may be one that is more recommended; the patient and the doctor work together so that the decision is well informed.

As your condition responds to treatment or changes, you and your doctor may also decide to make other adjustments as the situation warrants. Expect your chiropractic doctor to closely monitor your back pain so that you may be offered other chiropractic options from which to choose at a later date.

Tests: Just What the Doctor Ordered?

Tests ordered by your chiropractor should be based on a thorough understanding of your symptoms, condition, and necessity. The reasons for each test should be clear to you as well as how each test is done. The chiropractor should explain everything to you before having the test so that you feel comfortable and confident.

After the results are in, the chiropractor should go through them with you and discuss the findings in detail. In most cases, the doctor will show you the reports and explain to you what they mean.

Many tests result in a positive or negative where the relevance of each depends on the kind of test. The chiropractor should go through the positives and negatives with you and explain how they confirm any current or previous diagnoses. Before leaving his office, you should be clear on the test results and ready to move on to the treatment phase.

If you are currently on other treatments, the findings in your tests may indicate that a new form of treatment may be needed. This happens when something new is found that may be contributing to your back pain or if a previous condition has changed or worsened. Once you have all your test results, the treatment plan may be initiated.

As Your Treatment Progresses

From your first visit, to your final or less frequent maintenance visits, each individual experience is equally important. Your chiropractor wants to help you and ensure that your health is carefully monitored while in his care.

Your chiropractor will want to know if there are any changes, positive or negative, in your condition at each appointment, or if something changes unexpectedly between appointments. Always remember to report anything unusual regarding your back pain to your chiropractor immediately.

Make sure that you make every effort to follow the prescribed treatment as your chiropractic doctor has suggested. He wants to ensure that you are given the best possible care and that you are doing your part too. Especially since you and your doctor have worked out a treatment plan that has been mutually agreed upon and discussed. Your recovery from back pain may depend on it.

Common Diagnostic Tests

All About X-ray

A visit to the chiropractor or a medical doctor may include getting X-rays of your back and spine. This is a common test ordered by many chiropractors because it is a relatively simple way to get a quick thorough look at what may be causing or contributing to your back pain.

Most chiropractors are trained in X-ray technology and are very comfortable doing their own X-rays while some have specially trained staff in their office who do X-ray imaging. Since X-rays are excellent diagnostic tools for bones and vertebrae, they may be able to provide immediately useful information.

X-rays Defined

X-rays have been in use for more than one hundred years and are one of the most common imaging tests for diagnosing many conditions. The X-ray machine uses short wavelength energy beams that can penetrate almost anything except heavy metals.

They can provide good detail of the bone structure of the spine and include detailed images of vertebrae as well. Chiropractors may order X-rays to get a better view of your back and to detect other conditions such as instability of the spine, tumors, or fractures.

Evolution of The X-ray

The invention of X-ray imaging happened almost by accident in 1895 when a German physics professor named Wilhelm Roentgen was working with glass vacuum tubes and a cathode ray generator.

While working on his project, he noticed an unusual green light on the wall. The light was coming from the cathode ray generator and the path between the wall and the generator was blocked by various items in the room.

Roentgen quickly started placing more objects in front of the generator and again noticed the same result. It was when he was arranging other items that he noticed an outline of the bones from his hand on the wall. He did not know what to call this new kind of radiation ray, so he simply named it "X" to suggest that it was something unknown. To this day, his term "X" is included in this type of imaging as it is known as X-ray technology.

Many other advances have been made since Roentgen's groundbreaking work, but the basis for today's X-ray technique is largely attributed to this man's research and discovery.

How X-rays Work

X-rays are a form of electromagnetic radiation that penetrates through materials of light atoms. During an X-ray, an X-ray beam is sent through the body. Flesh and other soft tissue in the body can easily be penetrated by an X-ray beam. But bones contain varying amounts of calcium, and X-ray beams are not able to get through. The calcium blocks penetration of the X-ray beam. The image of bones seen on an X-ray is a shadow that appears on a film placed on the other side of the patient or object being X-rayed.

Because X-ray beams are most useful in images of bone, they do not provide as much detail in the soft tissue. For detailed images of organs, muscle, tendons, or discs in the back, MRI imaging is the preferred method. Chiropractors more frequently make use of X-rays because they work directly with bones and vertebrae found in the spine and are valuable diagnostic tools.

Using X-rays to Check Alignment of the Spine

X-rays can be used effectively for checking bone alignment by closely examining the shadows to determine if any of the bones in the spine do not appear aligned or if they are damaged. Misaligned bone structure may also be an indicator of instability in the spine.

If degeneration of the spine is suspected, an X-ray will show changes in the bone structure. The spaces between vertebrae may be increased or decreased depending on the reason for the abnormality. Evidence of bone spurs or other changes in joints and structure can also be seen in X-rays.

The Safety of X-rays

X-ray technology has come a long way since the invention of this now common imaging tool. The earliest X-ray machines exposed the patient to higher levels of radiation than the most modern machines in use today. New technological advances in medical imaging procedures have made the possibility of excessive radiation from X-rays almost impossible.

In fact, people are already exposed to varying amounts of radiation in day-to-day living from naturally occurring radioactive materials and cosmic radiation from outer space. The amounts are infinitely small and the amount of radiation from a plain X-ray does not amount to much more.

X-ray technicians are specially trained and experienced in X-ray technique and take all the necessary precautions to ensure that you are only exposed to the minimum amount of radiation. Patients are also generally given lead gowns as an added precaution to ensure even less possibility of exposure.

Since the benefits of having an X-ray far outweigh the possibility of any harm, most chiropractors are comfortable in using them to help diagnose conditions that may be causing your back pain.

All About MRI

MRI, or Magnetic Resonance Imaging, is a test that may be ordered by your chiropractor when there is a need for more detailed pictures of your back than is possible with an X-ray. An MRI can show even the smallest of abnormalities in tissue, organs, muscles or bones.

A chiropractor may want to confirm a suspected condition with MRI imaging because it is very useful in diagnosing back conditions where there is involvement with tissue or cartilage. It provides very detailed images of the discs in the back and surrounding tissue, which is very important in determining what is causing back pain.

What Is Magnetic Resonance Imaging?

It is a diagnostic tool used to take pictures of various parts of the body. The machine is usually quite large and the MRI scanner operates using a huge, high-powered magnet that rotates at great speed. The magnet works with radio waves and a scanner that is connected to a computer.

The computer is able to convert information from the MRI scanner into images. These images are produced in "cross-sectional" format where the part of the body being scanned looks like "slices" of small sections. The computer then arranges all of the "slices" into one larger image. It resembles an X-ray but shows more detail in the soft tissue.

The MRI scanner can also create three-dimensional images where an area may be viewed from virtually any angle. This is a very useful diagnostic tool, allowing the chiropractor to see any abnormality and how it is appears in relation to the entire area.

Why Order an MRI for Back Pain?

Many chiropractors will order an MRI for patients with back pain because it may give a clearer, more indicative picture of a problem due to its effectiveness in creating very detailed, specific images. Although X-rays are more common and less expensive, an MRI can get accurate pictures at different angles of more than just bones and joints.

In cases where the back pain is caused by soft tissue damage, an MRI can make it much clearer and easier to diagnose and treat conditions. When muscles and cartilage contribute to the back pain as well as does the spine, an MRI can show how all of these affect the patient, which gives a much better diagnostic tool for determining treatment.

Due to its specificity and detail, a chiropractor may decide that an MRI is needed to detect any condition or other reason for your back pain in its early stages. That is, if your back pain has been a fairly recent symptom, an MRI may be able to show an abnormality in your back regardless of how minor, and early detection may mean more success in treating it.

Features and Limitations of MRI Testing

Features   Many healthcare professionals tout the MRI as one of the greatest technological advances in diagnostic testing today. It provides great detail and can be used to confirm or check for a wide range of ailments. Due to its extremely fine-tuned imaging process, an MRI can show the size, shape, kind, and even three-dimensional view of practically any physical abnormality in the human body.

Getting an MRI is easy, generally non-invasive, and painless. There is usually no preparation needed for the test. This means that you are not required to change your food intake, medications, or regular activity in anticipation of your MRI.

MRI testing is also considered safe and uses natural forces. At no time are you exposed to radiation and there are no known harmful side effects.

All that is required is to report approximately 15 minutes early as you may need to put on a hospital gown and remove any jewelry, coins, or accessories before entering the MRI machine.

A Few Limitations   You may not be able to have MRI testing if you:

- ❖ Have a pacemaker
- ❖ Have steel or metal implants
- ❖ Have cochlear implants
- ❖ Use a neuro-stimulator
- ❖ Have an implanted drug-infusion device
- ❖ Are pregnant or think you might be pregnant

Some people are distracted by the loud noise of the magnets during MRI testing. This is only a minor limitation and is handled well by most people. If you are sensitive to noise, take a pair of earplugs with you and ask if you have permission to use them. Some MRI facilities can pipe in music to reduce the noise of the magnets.

One of the key requirements when having an MRI is that you must remain perfectly still for the entire testing session. This is usually not difficult for most adults, but may be slightly more difficult for children depending on the length of the MRI testing.

Depending on the number of areas to be tested with the MRI, a typical session may last up to one hour. Most patients understand that the MRI is designed to take thorough images and are willing to cooperate completely in this diagnostic process. In fact, some people are able to fall asleep during MRI testing!

The cost of an MRI is much more expensive than an X-ray or CAT scan. At times, an MRI will only be ordered if there is a specific reason or condition that warrants it.

In Conclusion   Overall, many patients seeking relief from back pain might very well be advised by their chiropractor to have an MRI. The advantages of this excellent diagnostic tool truly outweigh the disadvantages, especially since an MRI may be able to provide the necessary information to accurately assess and help your chiropractor treat your back pain.

Exercise Is Effective When Treating Back Pain, But Is It Right for You?

Back pain is a common problem among people of all shapes, sizes, ages, and professions.

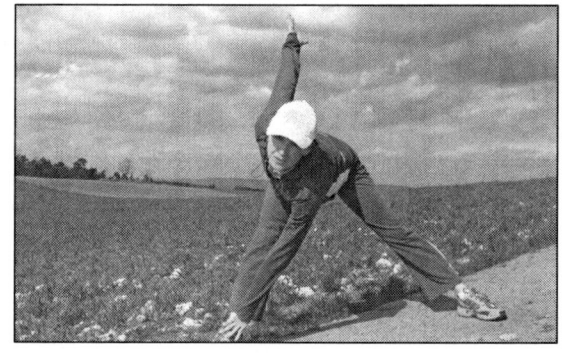

A variety of conservative treatment options is available to help avoid invasive procedures that involve surgery. For example, taking yoga classes to manage back pain is an example of using a conservative method to alleviate pain and even prevent future injury.

It is important to remember that physical therapy is an active treatment. The key difference between active and passive remedies is that passive treatments are being performed on a patient rather than a patient performing them. Medication, for instance, passively treats muscle pain.

Massage is another passive treatment. While massage therapists say that regular massages can help strengthen muscle, this form of treatment is still considered passive because patients are not active participants in the therapy.

Meanwhile, with active physical therapy, patients must practice self-discipline. It is always important to take responsibility for your health. Exercise usually requires a willingness to follow the program independently. For example, you may attend physical therapy sessions but also be assigned exercises to complete at home.

Or, if you are using exercise as a means of preventing future injury and improving your overall condition, you may take classes at a local health club, which certainly takes discipline. Most importantly, before beginning any exercise program, patients should always consult a physician. Doing so will ensure that the regimen is suited for the type of back pain you have.

Most people do not put much thought into the type of muscle pain they experience. There are different types of back pain, and the types will help determine which active therapy you rely upon for healing.

Acute Back Pain: Mixture of Rest and Exercise Is Best

The earliest phase of back pain is called the acute phase and lasts less than one month. This type of pain typically occurs in the lower back with most descriptions ranging from sharp pain to dull ache, and many patients report that they feel the pain more intensely on one side than the other.

Though exercise is beneficial in regaining flexibility and strengthening muscles, it is not recommended during the initial phase of acute back pain. Since injuries such as strained muscles usually cause acute back pain, it is best not to overexert the weakened muscle. Moreover, there is a good chance that surrounding muscles will compensate for the injured area; thus, these muscles are at risk for injury.

Instead, most physicians recommend a short period of rest during the initial phase of acute back pain. This resting period should last no longer than two days in order to prevent muscle loss. Moreover, back pain, especially if it is recurrent or chronic, has been shown to trigger depression in some patients.

Too much rest only adds to the potential for lack of motivation, which is just the opposite of what is necessary for recovery. In addition, physicians also recommend utilization of passive therapies such as hot and cold therapies, medication, and massage during the initial phase of acute back pain.

Subacute Back Pain

After the first couple of days, physical activity should be re-established. Furthermore, once the first five days have ended, the initial phase of acute back pain is finished. The acute phase in its entirety lasts less than a month and becomes subacute back pain, which lasts one to three months.

During the acute and sub-acute phases, patients are typically allowed to begin exercises programs. Of course, jogging and high-impact aerobics are still out of the question. Instead, you will be better served in continuing basic daily activities with some caution and incorporating low-impact exercise like walking.

Just remember to wear supportive shoes and avoid walking on pavement when possible. If there are grassy areas, for instance, walk in those places. Softer ground means less impact on joints. If you are unable or are otherwise uninterested in outdoor exercises, it is also safe to use stationary equipment such as a treadmill, bicycle, or elliptical machine. In addition, mild stretching exercises should be practiced to improve flexibility.

Exercise Is Essential for Alleviating Chronic and Recurrent Acute Back Pain

Whereas acute back pain is most often brought on by injury, chronic back pain takes hold in the nervous system and lasts more than three months. Researchers have found that exercise is more helpful in alleviating chronic back pain than acute and subacute back pain.

Physical activity has several benefits when it comes to treating lower back pain. First, many exercises improve flexibility, which is vital in relieving chronic back pain. When muscles are too tight, the spine is imbalanced and even simple movements can be very uncomfortable. Stretching frees tightened muscles and restores mobility.

Additionally, stabilization exercises like Pilates and yoga, for instance, help strengthen core muscles and keep the spine in a neutral position. Moreover, strong muscles do not strain or become fatigued as easily. And finally, low-impact aerobic activities condition and strengthen muscles. This keeps the spine balanced and prevents injury.

Not only is aerobic exercise good for muscles, it is beneficial overall. As mentioned, patients with chronic back pain may also become patients diagnosed with depression. However, exercise has also been proven to increase serotonin, a neurotransmitter in the brain that acts as a natural antidepressant. It is important to remember that passive conservative treatments such as hot and cold therapies, medication, and massage therapy may be utilized when managing chronic back pain, in addition to chiropractic treatments.

On the other hand, recurrent acute back pain typically occurs when the acute pain previously experienced by a patient flares up again. Most patients have at least one repeated incident of acute back pain. The best way to prevent this from happening is to strengthen and condition the muscles.

Since weak muscles are strained easier than well-conditioned ones, exercise is an integral part of preventing recurrent acute back pain. However, if you encounter this problem, it is best to follow the same pattern as before, taking a brief period of rest and then carefully adding stretching and conditioning exercises to your routine.

Moreover, if you have a hobby or occupation that is hard on your muscles and joints, additional support may be necessary. For example, if you work in a place that requires a lot of lifting, it is wise to wear a lifting belt. This back brace, often made of cloth or canvas, assists muscles that would otherwise become fatigued and easily strained.

From Stretching to Strengthening: How Active Therapies Relieve Back Pain

While most passive therapies treat the symptoms of back pain, active physical therapy corrects problems causing muscle strain, inflammation, and a host of other conditions that make back pain unbearable. Active physical therapy is an effective conservative treatment for recurrent back pain.

When back pain is recurrent, it is most likely prompted by certain strenuous activities. Of course, muscle tension and strain is also brought on by less obvious factors like poor posture or unhealthy sleeping positions. Fortunately, there are several active physical therapies from which to choose. Your chiropractor can help you determine the type of exercise most appropriate for the phase of pain you are experiencing.

Specific Rest

This form of treatment involves controlled exercises specified by a chiropractor or physical therapist. During specific rest, patients must avoid the activity that caused the muscle strain or other injury. However, they should perform controlled exercises in order to regain mobility and range of motion in addition to maintaining muscle strength. In some cases, physicians prescribe braces that may or may not be used during exercises, usually performed several times a day.

Stretching and Increased Flexibility

Muscles that are too tight can lead to unhealthy imbalances in the spine. When muscles constrict motion, the spinal movements are imbalanced, which causes back pain. Imbalanced movement may also cause injury. Performing stretching exercises increases flexibility and helps prevent injury and even re-injury.

Though it may take time for this treatment method to produce results, stretching is also very effective for treating chronic back pain. This is true because stretching provides prolonged relief that can only be experienced with increased freedom of movement. There are specific muscles that should be targeted when doing this type of exercise.

First of all, stretching the hamstrings, which are located at the back of the legs, can help minimize lower back pressure. Hamstrings assist gluteus muscles and hip flexors. Moreover, the gluteus muscles should be stretched because they support the pelvis as well as hip flexibility.

The Psoas Major is another muscle that may have a major role in lower back pain. Since it is attached to the front of the spine, an overly-tightened Psoas Major can make prolonged standing or kneeling intolerable. And finally, the Piriformis, running from the back of the thigh bone to the base of the spine, can produce sciatica-like pain when it is too tight. It has even been associated with sacroiliac joint dysfunction.

Stabilization and Strengthening Exercises

Muscles running along the spine, particularly back and abdominal muscles, are vital because they support movements occurring throughout the body. These muscles often referred to as "core" muscles provide important stability for the spine.

When these muscles are weak, even simple daily tasks can place unhealthy stresses on the spine, which often leads to back pain. Of course, there are exercises that focus on the body's core, Pilates, for example. Since Pilates strengthens core muscles, it supports good posture, which is a very basic need for maintaining a healthy spine. Not only does it increase strength in weak core muscles, it also encourages flexibility. In fact, many physical therapy routines include Pilates because it is a form of exercise that does not require a great deal of physical exertion; therefore, the risk of injury or further damage is minimal.

Furthermore, dynamic lumbar stabilization and McKenzie extension exercises are also recommended for patients hoping to strengthen back muscles. Dynamic lumbar stabilization first helps patients find the position that is most comfortable, which is called the "neutral spine." Then, exercises help back muscles maintain that position and also help the patients remain more aware of it. McKenzie extension exercises, on the other hand, are designed to reduce pain from a degenerated or herniated disk. In many cases, these exercises relieve pain in the back and legs.

Low-Impact Aerobics

In aerobic exercise, low impact refers to exercise that does not involve a lot of jumping, running or any other movements that pound on the joints. For example, water aerobics provide all the cardiovascular and strengthening benefits of aerobics with very minimal impact on joints.

Aerobic exercise also helps with muscle coordination and conditioning. Muscles have to be trained to work together so that one muscle or group does not have to over-compensate for the other. This helps keep physical activity under control, preventing re-injury. Thus, it is best to focus on total body fitness rather than just treating one specific area.

Moreover, conditioning is very beneficial in preventing any type of back pain.

When a patient engages in aerobic activity, the muscles receive more oxygen and circulation is improved. Increased oxygen levels help muscles to move fluidly and continuously. In contrast, less oxygen only encourages muscles to move in spurts, creating a potential risk for injury. Of course, it is important to pace yourself when starting and implementing a conditioning program. Overexerting the body and re-injuring muscles will only set you back further.

Exercises Should Be Monitored by Your Doctor or Chiropractor

When treating back pain, a physician should always be consulted beforehand. While this is true with any treatment option, exercises should be handled with extra caution. Doing exercises that are too strenuous or inappropriate for the muscle's condition could make the injury worse; thus, the pain would only increase. Chiropractors and physical therapists have the ability to evaluate back pain and its cause. Because of their expertise, they have the tools to assign the most effective and safest treatment options to a given condition.

Take Initiative and Responsibility for Your Back Health: The Best Aerobic Exercises for Back Pain Relief

While stretching, stabilization and strengthening are all beneficial in relieving back pain, conditioning exercises help to relief chronic back pain and achieve total body fitness. As stated before, it is essential to keep back muscles in shape in order to keep them from becoming fatigued and strained. Also keeping your entire body fit lessens your risk of back injury.

For example, when a person is overweight, the extra pounds place unnecessary stress on the joints, including those along the spine. As the body becomes unbalanced from extra weight, back muscles are forced to work harder than they are able. First and foremost, the body is not prepared to carry the extra weight. In addition, muscles are weak, out of shape, and vulnerable to injury.

When incorporating a new conditioning program into your lifestyle, it is imperative to comply with all the conditioning recommendations and be prepared to follow the program independently. For instance, if a physician suggests half an hour of low-impact aerobic activity per day, the patient must make an honest attempt to complete the workout.

A new conditioning program may translate to more pain at first. Typically, muscles are increasingly sore one or two days after the program begins. However, patients with self-discipline soon find that the sore muscles strengthen and their pain tolerance increases as they remain committed to the exercise program.

It is essential to pace yourself, increasing the activity as you become stronger. For example, your physician may prescribe only 20 minutes of water aerobics per session, but you can build up to the average time of 45 minutes as you continue to benefit from the training.

Though patients with chronic back pain often see the most dramatic results from total body conditioning, this type of program can be appropriate no matter what stage of back pain you are experiencing. The key is to find the style of workout that is best for your body. There are many different exercise programs available. Some are right outside your front door and others are offered by local health clubs. Here are a few of the different conditioning exercises that help alleviate back pain.

Outdoor Activities: Walking and Cycling

Both these activities make great outdoor hobbies. For those who enjoy being outside, walking or cycling routines begin right outside your door. Of course, if the air-conditioned comfort of a gym is preferred, treadmills and stationary bicycles offer the same conditioning advantages.

The most important points to consider are the advantages to those who want relief for back pain. Walking and cycling are great cardiovascular exercises; they burn calories and contribute to overall weight loss. Patients benefit from the increased circulation, which helps detoxify the muscles. Furthermore, enhanced oxygen levels reduce muscle pain. Brisk walking helps improve posture, increase flexibility, and even reduce the risk of osteoporosis.

Aqua Aerobics

If you have a swimming pool, this program may be as convenient as your backyard. If not, there is no reason to be discouraged. Many local health clubs offer water aerobics classes several times a week. Since approximately 90 percent of a person's body weight is supported by the water, this is one of the best workouts when it comes to minimizing impact on the joints. In fact, it nearly eliminates impact.

Water provides resistance to movements, which helps strengthen muscles. Like traditional aerobics, water aerobics works on the entire body, making this form of exercise useful for those striving toward total body fitness. During a typical session, participants burn about 500 to 700 calories.

Also, patients enjoy improved circulation and thus pain relief. Contrary to popular belief, being a good swimmer is not necessary because participants are only asked to exercise in water that is chest deep. People who are unable to swim should take comfort in the fact that many aqua aerobics instructors are certified lifeguards. At the YMCA, for example, instructors are certified and there is usually another lifeguard outside the pool.

Swimming

Lap swimming has many of the same benefits as aqua aerobics. Swimming conditions muscles from the shoulders down to muscles in your feet. Swimming also keeps the body cool. In fact, you will not even feel sweat. Like water aerobics, swimming eliminates any impact on the body's joints. The water provides resistance and allows for a total body workout, strengthening the muscles and increasing the heart rate.

In truth, swimming can be just as strenuous as running or jogging but without the pounding that often causes discomfort in joints. Still, there are a few precautions beginners should take when starting a swimming exercise program.

First, when doing a front stroke (usually called freestyle), it is important not to hyperextend the arms. Additionally, swimming requires you to turn your head in order to breathe. The problem here is the potential for strain and fatigue in neck muscles.

There are several ways to avoid this complication. One of the easiest ways is to swim with a floatation device such as a noodle. This keeps your head above the surface, allowing you to look forward and breathe naturally. Using a snorkel also helps by permitting you to keep your head down and your spine aligned. If you prefer to swim without a floatation device, simply limit the amount of times you turn to breathe. While many beginning swimmers take a breath with every other stroke, you may find success in breathing every three or five strokes.

Active Therapies: The Exercise Tools You Need for a Well-Rounded Workout

Active physical therapy often provides the most effective relief for patients suffering from back pain. For those with acute back pain and certainly those with chronic back pain, physical therapy offers several important benefits. For example, a patient with acute back pain will benefit from increased circulation. Better circulation helps ease the pain by supplying muscles with increased oxygen and nutrients.

Acute back pain typically requires a short rest period. Furthermore, patients with chronic back pain are most likely to see results with an exercise program. These programs encourage total body fitness, which means lower weight and stronger muscles.

There are several different types of conditioning programs available for patients with lower back pain.

Aerobic activity is not the only ingredient to an effective exercise routine. Stretching and strengthening are also very important. For instance, before your workout begins, it is pivotal to practice a stretching routine. Stretching increases flexibility and allows the muscles to warm up before more strenuous activity begins. Additionally, exercises like abdominal crunches are a great way to build up trunk muscles.

The Swiss Ball is highly recommended by chiropractors and doctors. While many people use an exercise ball for several areas of the body, people with back pain find it especially useful as part of their stretching and strengthening routines.

The Swiss Ball: A Tool for Balance and Stability

The Swiss Ball is commonly prescribed as part of an active physical therapy program in order to alleviate lower back pain. Rather than performing exercises on the hard floor, patients have the option of using a Swiss Ball to provide comfort and strengthen muscles at the same time.

In fact, this tool allows you to focus on your back and abdominal muscles, which are often referred to as core muscles. When all of the back and abdominal muscles are strong, it helps the spine to remain balanced and stable; thus, your body is not relying on only a few muscles to do all the work.

You do not have to use the Swiss Ball just for exercise to realize all its benefits. In fact, many physical therapists recommend using this device instead of an office chair for a couple of hours each day. It helps the body use back and abdominal muscles more than a chair, which strengthens muscles of the back and abdomen and even improves posture.

Moreover, by rolling around on the ball (perhaps going from the desk to the file cabinet), you stay mobile, which eases the pain caused by stiff muscles. Of course, the Swiss Ball is ideal for stretching exercises and strengthening exercises for the abdominal muscles. Here are a couple of the most common training techniques:

Lower Back Stretch

Stretching the back muscles helps to increase flexibility, which makes movement more comfortable and prevents muscle strain in the future. In order to perform this exercise, lie face down over the exercise ball, placing it beneath the abdomen. Allow your arms and legs to wrap around the ball but keep them relaxed. Your knees will go to the floor and your hands will gently hold the exercise ball. This stretch curves your back, letting the back muscles gently stretch while providing support.

Side-to-Side Stretch

This stretching exercise works on the back as well as the abdominal muscles. Simply lie on your back with your knees bent and your calves resting on the exercise ball. Also, rest both arms at your sides with the palms on the floor. Slowly turn the legs to one side as far as possible. It is essential to stretch as far as you can without slipping off of the exercise ball or feeling any pain. Then, return to the starting position and repeat on the other side.

Abdominal Crunches

Since abdominal muscles also support the spine, keeping them in shape will help prevent back pain. For instance, healthy posture is very important to maintaining a balanced spine. Strong core muscles keep help ensure stability. To complete this exercise, lie on your back with your knees bent and your feet elevated on a chair or table. You may cross your hands on your chest or rest them behind your head. Finally, gradually raise your shoulders and upper back off of the exercise ball. Then slowly descend and repeat as needed.

Same Shape, Different Sizes: Which Is Best for You?

For patients with lower back pain, chiropractors typically recommend a large exercise ball. Of course, the best way to make sure it is the right size for your body is to size it according to your height. The general rule of thumb is:

> Fifty-five centimeters for those less than 5 feet tall
>
> Sixty-five centimeters ranging from 5 feet to 5 feet 7 inches
>
> Seventy-five cm ranging from 5 feet 8 inches to 6 feet 2 inches
>
> Eighty-five centimeters for those over 6 feet 2 inches tall

Though sizing the Swiss Ball is very important, it is also imperative that you keep the ball well inflated. Furthermore, as with any exercise, you should consult a physician before adding a Swiss Ball to your workout routine. A healthcare professional can help determine how much exercise is best for the type of back pain you are experiencing.

Additionally, as any healthcare professional will suggest, it is essential not to overdo any type of physical training. In fact, there are strength coaches who have publicly criticized the exercise ball because so many patients have a tendency to overuse it. Of course, this only leads to strained and fatigued muscles, defeating the purpose altogether. Thus, patients must be responsible for their treatments, performing the exercises as prescribed but not overexerting.

Conditioning Exercises: Maximize Your Aerobic Activity and Minimize Back Pain

One of the most misunderstood aspects of treating back pain is the importance of physical activity, particularly aerobic activity. By now, you have learned that physical activity is vital in strengthening, conditioning, and increasing flexibility of the muscles. Moreover, you are probably well aware that strong, well-conditioned muscles are less susceptible to fatigue and strain, which can mean permanent relief from chronic back pain in most patients.

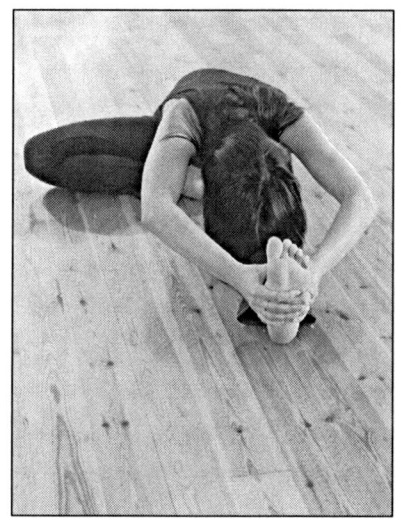

Still, most of the conditioning exercises that patients think of as beneficial are those that focus directly on the muscles. What you may not know is the significance of exercising one of the most important muscles in the human body, the heart. This is the key difference between muscle exercises and aerobic activity.

For example, there are specific exercises designed to encourage flexibility and strength to a specific muscle or muscle group. In addition to these benefits, aerobic activity provides a cardiovascular workout along with advantages that are unique to this type of training.

For instance, aerobic activity improves circulation and oxygen absorbed by the muscles. It also encourages the production of endorphins, which act as a natural antidepressant and create an overall sense of happiness. Most importantly, it increases the patient's metabolic rate, which can be defined as the number of calories your body burns per day. Nevertheless, this helps to treat obesity, an epidemic of modern society that contributes significantly to the condition of back pain.

Although most people are aware that obesity can lead to heart problems, hypertension, diabetes, and colon cancer. And most patients who are overweight make the connection that the extra pounds create unnecessary work for the spine. However, what most of them do not consider is the fact that being overweight can worsen symptoms associated with osteoarthritis, osteoporosis, spinal stenosis, spondylolisthesis, and degenerative disc disease.

Additionally, it can lead to sciatica, which occurs when excessive pressure is placed on the sciatic nerve and is characterized by a shooting pain in the lower back and leg. Thus, extra weight compromises the natural structure of the spine and can become damaging. This is true because the spine is designed not only to carry the body's weight but also to distribute it evenly.

When there is extra weight, particularly around the waist, this forces the spine to adjust in very unnatural, unhealthy ways. The lower back is especially vulnerable to damage. Additional weight in the midsection, combined with weak muscles in the pelvis, back and legs, may pull the pelvis forward, causing an abnormal curve in the spine.

In spite of all the complications obesity can cause, aerobic exercise enables patients to fight back against obesity and regain their healthy, mobile, and reasonably pain-free lives.

There are numerous aerobic activities from which to choose (walking, biking, water aerobics, and swimming, to name a few). Nevertheless, what most have yet to learn is that there are simple techniques that help to maximize any conditioning program. Here are a few ways to get the most out of your aerobic training program:

Choose Wisely

When deciding upon an activity, there are a few factors to consider. First, do your best to select an activity you already enjoy. If you like the calm, quiet workout that only lap swimming can provide, sign up for a membership at your local YMCA. If you love the outdoors, find a nice walking or biking trail.

If you tend to become bored easily, you will be better served if you add some variety to your weekly workout plan. For example, bike every Monday, swim every Wednesday and take a nature hike every Friday. Whichever exercise you choose, you must also make sure that you can perform it for 20 minutes or longer. Since it can take about 20 minutes for your heart rate to reach its fullest potential, it is essential that the activity continue for at least that long in order to facilitate calorie burning.

Pace Yourself: Gradual Increase Produces Long-Term Results

Though it can be difficult to resist, it is always best to pace yourself in every aspect of your exercise routine. For instance, you should begin each session with approximately 10 minutes of stretching and then follow the stretching with a warm-up period. Furthermore, the warm-up period should last only about five minutes. Once the body is warmed up, you can intensify the workout.

While it is important to choose an activity that increases the metabolic rate and burns calories, it is also vital that you continue the activity long enough for it to serve its purpose. Since it takes at least 20 minutes for the heart rate to increase, this amount of time should be the minimum. Therefore, the best solution is to start with 20-minute workout sessions four to five times each week. Then, over a period of approximately 10 to 12 weeks, you can increase the sessions by five minutes each week. This should help you gradually build up to 60 minutes of aerobic activity four to five times each week.

Remember the Simple Details

One of the most important activities people take for granted is breathing. Sometimes when a person is bearing down and concentrating very hard on the task at hand, they forget to breathe.

Breathing should be elevated somewhat but panting is a sign that the workout is too strenuous. In addition to oxygen, the body needs water in order to get the maximum benefit from aerobic activity. Furthermore, water keeps muscles hydrated, which is important to prevent cramping. Also, water flushes out the body, making it more productive in all areas.

Brace Yourself: How Back Braces Relieve Pain and Prevent Injury

Many patients rely on back braces as a conservative treatment option to alleviate back pain. While many different back pain treatments focus on increasing movement and flexibility, there are occasions during which it may be necessary to immobilize areas of the spine. When a patient encounters back pain from an injury, for example, it may be essential to prevent movement in order to allow the damaged muscles to heal.

There is some risk of muscle loss if the area is immobilized for an extended period of time but the risk of re-injury can be worse. To effectively and safely control movement, nearly all physicians advocate the use of back braces. Moreover, many patients rely on back braces in addition to physical therapy or other passive therapies. Opportunely, there is a variety of neck and back braces available.

Trochanteric Belt

The Trochanteric Belt fits around the pelvis, between the trochanter, which is the bony portion below at the top of the thigh bone, and the iliac ridges or crests. Since this belt is placed across the pelvis and above the legs, it is useful in relieving lower back pain, particularly during pregnancy. During a study cited by chiroweb.com, fifty-four pregnant women were given a Trochanteric Belt to relieve their lower back pain. Of those fifty-four, thirty-nine were relieved of their symptoms.

Sacroiliac Belt

Sometimes referred to as a lumbrosacral belt, this back brace also helps stabilize the lower back. Furthermore, this type of belt immobilizes the area by compressing the joints between the hipbone and sacrum at the base of the spine. Most Sacroiliac Belts are approximately ten to fifteen or twenty to thirty centimeters wide and they are worn at a slightly higher position than trochanteric belts.

Corset

Corsets are available in a few different lengths. A short corset, for instance, is used for low back pain, while a longer one is used for damaged areas in the mid to lower thoracic spine. Though the stereotypical corset is one that women wore centuries ago to make their waists look smaller, modern corsets serve to relieve back pain. This kind of relief would most likely be impossible to imagine for women forced to wear the earlier corsets. Today, they are used to provide comfort and improve posture. In fact, some corsets are worn voluntarily by people who do a lot of heavy lifting because they help prevent painful muscle strain.

Rigid Braces

When the other back supports are not firm enough, physicians prescribe a rigid brace for low back pain and spinal instability. Williams Brace, for example, is a rigid brace that allows the patient to bend because it has no vertical pieces in the middle.

Meanwhile, the Chair-back Brace holds the lumbar spine in the neutral position, restricts sideways movements and limits rotation of the lower spine. And finally, the Raney Flexion Jacket keeps the lumbar spine in a neutral tilt, reducing curvature of the lumbar spine.

Even though rigid braces are arduous for some patients, they are useful in relieving lower back pain. Since rigid braces are often used for more severe injuries such as fractures, they play an important role in providing relief and preventing further injury. Of course, some patients complain that rigid braces weigh them down and make them feel too warm. Fortunately, patients are only required to wear them while standing and are instructed to removing them while lying down.

Hyperextension Brace

One main feature of hyperextension braces is that they have a rectangular metal frame in front; thus, pressure is placed over the breast bone as well as the pubic bone, which is conducive for extension of the spine. Physicians usually prescribe hyperextension braces to treat frontal compression fractures located where the thoracic and lumbar areas of the spine come together.

Additionally, since they restrict bending of the thoracic and lumbar spine, hyperextension braces are typically used after surgery for spinal fusion. Another important feature of this hyperextension brace is that it provides "three-point stabilization" to the spine through a front abdominal pad, a chest pad, and a rear pad strategically located at the level of the fracture.

Molded Jacket

The main purpose of the molded jacket is to spread pressure over a large area; thus, it is designed to remove excess pressure from overloaded or unstable areas by distributing pressure evenly. Since surrounding muscles can become irritated from overcompensating to make up for weak muscles, braces like the molded jacket are beneficial to patients with weak or strained muscles. Not only does the molded jacket alleviate back pain, it helps prevent new injuries that may only cause more discomfort for the patient in the future.

Lifting Belt

As mentioned, many people wear corsets in order to prevent muscle strain or re-injury while lifting heavy objects. Similarly, lifting belts are designed to reduce low-back strain and muscle fatigue from lifting heavy objects. Furthermore, lifting belts are soft because they are usually made of cloth or canvas with no stays.

It is important to remember that back pain can be treated and prevented with devices such as the lifting belt. When lifting heavy items repeatedly, it is easy for muscles to become fatigued; therefore, wearing a lifting belt to assist these muscles is a proactive way to treat back pain.

Psychological Dependency on Back Braces

Back braces come with numerous benefits. Not only are they used to treat existing back pain, they are helpful in preventing further injury as muscles and joint heal. Moreover, they even aid in the prevention of re-injury. Still, psychological addiction can occur in patients using back braces.

In such cases, even when a patient is restored to health, he or she feels dependent upon it for physical assistance. In a situation like this, it is important to heed the advice of physicians. They are trained and will know when it is best to discontinue using a brace.

If a brace is worn for too long, it could result in muscular atrophy, a condition in which muscles that are not used enough become too weak. As many people struggling with back pain already know, weak muscles are strained and injured easily. Of course, patients should consult their physicians both before and after treatment in order to ensure that they are using the correct brace and not using it longer than necessary.

Passive Therapies for Back Pain

B ack pain is, unfortunately, a part of everyday life for many of us. In fact, about 85% of the American population experience disabling low back pain at least once during the course of their lives. The problem of back pain is so widespread that one researcher estimates that, at any given time, approximately 6.8% of the adult United States population is suffering from an episode of back pain lasting more than two weeks.

It stands to reason that when one is in pain, the body's muscles become tense and less pliable. Therefore, chiropractors and other health professionals such as physical therapists have turned to passive therapies such as ultrasound to help relax tensed muscles. This type of soothing passive therapy enables the more active therapy such as manipulation and exercise to be more effective and pain-free.

Passive therapies are something that a chiropractor or physical therapist does to you. It is called passive because you don't really have to do anything. In this chapter we are going to discuss the most common passive physical therapy treatments.

The Therapeutic Benefits of Ultrasound Therapy

The use of ultrasound as a passive modality has long been employed by chiropractors and physical therapists alike. It is widely accepted as the best form of heat treatment for soft tissue injuries. But what is ultrasound therapy and how does it work?

First, let us investigate the ultrasound equipment itself. Consisting of a high-frequency generator and a wand-like applicator, an ultrasound machine utilizes sound (ultrasonic) waves, which are transmitted to injured soft tissues and surrounding blood vessels.

When ultrasound therapy is applied directly to the skin, a slow, circular motion is utilized. This process can implement a water-based gel or can even take place under water when the area being treated is an irregular surface, such as the ankle. Normally, the depth of ultrasound wave penetration is about five centimeters.

As the ultrasonic waves are absorbed, tissue molecules begin to vibrate creating the effect of a microscopic massage. This vibrating massage gradually converts into thermal heat, which relaxes and warms muscles and ligaments prior to more active treatment. The heat created by ultrasound also promotes vascular dilation thereby increasing beneficial blood flow to an injured area.

Ultrasound therapy can be administered up to five times per week, depending upon the attending health professional's treatment plan. A typical ultrasound session will last about eight minutes for each area being treated.

Two Very Different Methods of Ultrasound

Ultrasound passive therapy can utilize either a continuous or a pulsed setting. Each method has a very specific targeted use.

There is evidence from randomized trials that *low-intensity pulsed ultrasound treatment* may significantly reduce the length of time required for fractures to properly heal. This is of particular importance in light of the fact that approximately 5% to 10% of the 5.6 million fractures that occur annually in the United States experience delayed healing.

Continuous ultrasound therapy is the more typically utilized type of ultrasound administered by chiropractors and physical therapists, as their area of specialty usually involves muscles and ligaments. The soothing, deep heat of continuous ultrasound therapy has been shown to be beneficial in the relief of pain and soft tissue inflammation.

Of particular benefit are conditions such as chronic low back pain, tennis elbow, shoulder impingement, muscle sprains, strains or spasms, and joint stiffness. Many times, depending upon the treatment area, range of motion is significantly increased as a result of this passive form of treatment.

Ultrasound Is Not "One Size Fits All"

Unfortunately, ultrasound therapy does not constitute an effective modality for every patient. For example, patients with acute infections or with a tendency to hemorrhage are not suitable candidates for ultrasound. Nor are patients who are pregnant or under six years of age. Additionally, the presence of occlusive vascular disease, blood clots, fractures, or a previous laminectomy all precludes the use of ultrasound therapy.

Additionally, a study by the National Institutes of Health found that patients suffering from lumbar disk herniation may not respond well to ultrasound therapy. In two case studies, this research found that the application of ultrasound to the lumbar paraspinal region increased, rather than reduced, pain in a radiating pattern.

Ultrasound Paired with Manipulation

Ultrasound therapy provides a passive approach to pain control and reduction of inflammation. But it is not a "stand-alone" form of treatment and should never serve as a substitute for more active therapy, such as spinal manipulation and prescribed exercise. To do so puts a patient at significant risk of a more serious injury and increased pain. Simply because the injured muscle or ligament feels better after an ultrasound treatment does not indicate that the soft tissue has healed.

The fact is that ultrasound is only a part of the treatment puzzle. For proper healing and optimum pain relief, it must be combined with other forms of more active treatment.

Paired with professional chiropractic care, for example, ultrasound therapy can be particularly beneficial. By first relaxing painfully tense muscles, the body becomes much more receptive to spinal manipulation. Additionally, ultrasound relaxes the affected area's blood vessels, which increases blood flow. This increased blood flow carries vital oxygen to stressed or injured soft tissues, encouraging and speeding the healing process.

During the course of a spinal manipulation, a skilled chiropractor locates spine and nerve stress caused by vertebrae impinging spinal nerves and then gently and painlessly realigns specific vertebrae, thus releasing pressure on nerves and body structures.

Overall, ultrasound therapy is a very effective and soothing form of passive therapy when addressing back pain. However, it should only be administered by a licensed healthcare provider or by a trained therapist under the supervision of a professional healthcare provider. And, remember, the inclusion of treatment by a qualified chiropractor or other health professional is key to proper recovery from injury and pain.

Massage Therapy — A Soothing Touch for Back Pain

If you are one of the many millions of people who frequently suffer from back pain, massage may just be the soothing touch you have been searching for.

Long considered a luxury rather than a legitimate therapy, massage has truly come into its own in the last several years. In fact, a university research team found that massage lessens lower back pain, depression, and anxiety, and even improves sleep.[1] Many healthcare providers now include massage as a beneficial addition to traditional treatment of lower back pain.

Massage therapy offers a number of very tangible health benefits, such as improved blood circulation, muscle relaxation, increased range of motion, and increased endorphin levels.

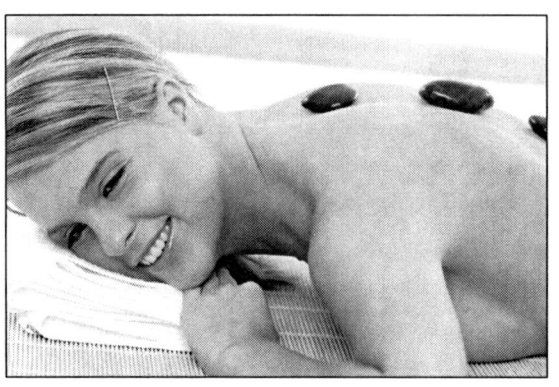

Interestingly, this increased level of endorphin is quite possibly one of the strongest benefits gained through massage therapy. Endorphins are natural pain relieving substances created by the body. With a chemical structure similar to morphine, this natural analgesic is extremely effective in the management of chronic pain.

Combining Massage Therapy with Chiropractic

Massage therapy, regardless of the type of massage chosen, will produce the most beneficial results when it is part of a treatment plan that incorporates chiropractic manipulation. The reason for this is simple: although massage therapy provides fast relief of back pain, it does not address the root problem actually causing the pain.

Massage therapy can be incredibly effective in preparing the body to receive optimum benefit from chiropractic manipulation, but simply cannot replace the health benefits achieved via professional spinal realignment.

Which Type of Massage Is Best for You?

Therapeutic massage has helped millions of people escape from the agony of back pain, even if only temporarily. It can relieve muscle tension, spasms, aches, stiffness and inflammation. Yet how do you decide which form of massage therapy will best address your back pain?

Here is a quick overview of the most common forms of massage:

Trigger point myotherapy   Also called neuromuscular massage therapy, this is likely the most effective type of massage therapy for lower back pain caused by soft tissue

[1]International Journal of Neuroscience, 106, 131–145

injury. Trigger points are typically found in tight bands of muscle and can radiate pain to other areas of the body. With trigger point myotherapy, alternating levels of direct pressure are concentrated on the area of a painful muscle spasm. The muscle is also gently stretched at the same time.

An interesting factoid about trigger point myotherapy is that it has had a very famous patient. Before he became President of the United States, a young Senator John F. Kennedy suffered from such debilitating back pain that he missed nearly three-fourths of the votes from the Senate floor. A physician treated this pain with remarkable success by locating the tender spot in the muscle (the trigger point) that was sending pain to another part of Kennedy's body.

Myofascial release   Myofascial release massage releases the tension from the fibrous bands of tissue that connect and support muscles. This fibrous tissue is referred to as fascia. Using a gentle, kneading massage to stretch, lengthen, soften, and realign these bands of tissue, myofascial release is often a very effective massage therapy after a muscle injury.

Deep tissue massage   This form of massage is very effective in releasing chronic muscle tension by applying deep, direct pressure and slow strokes *across* the grain of the muscle rather than *with* the grain as is used in myofascial release. Deep tissue massage can help break down and eliminate binding scar tissue, while also releasing toxins from muscle and promoting enhanced circulation.

Shiatsu   Shiatsu is a modern massage therapy deeply rooted in traditional Oriental medicine. Its principles are similar to acupuncture, but does not utilize needles. Shiatsu combines both pressure and stretching techniques, similar to trigger point myotherapy. This type of massage stimulates circulation while also releasing both toxins and tension from the muscles, allowing the patient to achieve a deep state of relaxation.

Swedish massage   Swedish massage is, undoubtedly, the most well-known type of massage. Using firm but gentle pressure and long, gliding strokes, it improves circulation, eases muscle tension and pain, improves flexibility and creates an overall sense of relaxation.

What Should You Expect After Massage Therapy?

Problematic muscles that were causing back pain should be noticeably more relaxed following massage therapy. If you received trigger point myotherapy, any initial soreness following the massage should fade after about twenty-four hours.

Muscles should remain relaxed for between four and fourteen days, depending, of course, on your level of stress, activity, and severity of back pain before the massage therapy.

A Word of Caution

If painful back muscles do not begin to relax in response to massage therapy, it is quite likely that inflammation is present. Massage is typically not the best treatment for inflamed muscles. Instead, you should seek out a professional chiropractor for treatment of the inflammation.

How to Find A Massage Therapist Who Is Right for You

First, talk to other people who have received massage therapy. Ask about their experiences with massage therapy. It is infinitely wiser to be referred to a massage therapist by someone who has had good personal success with a specific therapist than to simply pick a name out of the telephone book.

Also ask your chiropractor for the name of any recommended massage therapists.

Another great referral resource is the American Massage Therapy Association (http://www.amtamasssage.org/). This is a worldwide association, so regardless of where you live, chances are this organization can refer you to a qualified massage therapist in your area.

Transcutaneous Electrical Nerve Stimulation: A New Twist to an Ancient Therapy

Electricity has been used in one form or another for many thousands of years. For example, unearthed evidence indicates that ancient Egyptian healers often utilized electric fish to relieve pain. In ancient Greece, sufferers of arthritis and headaches apparently received similar treatment, with archeological finds indicating that electrogenic torpedo fish were used to relieve pain. In the 16th century through the 18th century, ingenious devices which created static electricity were used for the treatment of headaches and various other pains. In fact, Benjamin Franklin was a well-known proponent of electric stimulation as an effective form of pain relief.

Today, transcutaneous electrical nerve stimulation, also referred to simply as TENS, is a widely accepted form of pain relief. TENS therapy is a passive, non-invasive form of treatment that typically has no side effects. Unlike pain medication, it has no potential for addiction and appears to be effective in the reduction of both acute and chronic pain.

How Does TENS Work?

There are several theories about how the controlled application of low-voltage electricity works to relieve pain. Many healthcare providers propose that such application affects the nerves, which perceive pain, while others believe that it interferes with normal nerve pathways. Another theory is that transcutaneous (which means "applied via the skin") electrical nerve stimulation encourages the production of endorphins, a natural pain-killer chemical produced by the body.

A typical battery-operated TENS unit consists of a portable pulse generator, a small transformer and frequency and intensity controls. This form of pain relief therapy is delivered via electrodes strategically attached to various areas of the body. The specific sites where these electrode pads are placed, along with the frequency and intensity of the current, are crucial factors in achieving optimal results.

Available only by prescription, a conventional TENS unit is about the size of a cigarette pack. It is completely portable and worn around the waist, allowing the wearer to turn it on or off to maintain the desired level of pain management.

Three Different Forms of TENS

Conventional TENS   This form of electric current therapy involves the use of high-frequency, low-intensity current applied on or near painful areas of the body. Relief usually begins within just a few minutes of initiating TENS stimulation, but the pain relief also typically disappears within a few seconds after the machine is turned off. So, to maximize the benefits of this type of passive therapy, it is necessary for the TENS unit to be used for long periods throughout the day.

Electroacupuncture   Also known as EAP, electroacupuncture is a unique blend of electric stimulation therapy and acupuncture. Developed by the Chinese in the 1950s, this method of pain management was initially used as a surgical anesthesia. It requires that acupuncture needles outfitted with flexible wires be placed at specific trigger points. These wires are attached to a pulse generator. Pulses of high-intensity electrical current are applied to the needles, stimulating the nerves at the acupuncture point.

Acupuncture-like TENS (ALTENS)   This form of pain relief therapy is also applied at acupuncture trigger points, but without acupuncture needles. Instead, as is the application method with conventional TENS, electrode pads are affixed to the skin. Acupuncture-like TENS is generally considered a safer method of treatment than electro-acupuncture, simply because the risk of infection from needles is eliminated. Additionally, ALTENS is much less likely to cause bruising or organ damage.

Typically, it is necessary to increase the intensity of the electric stimulation when ALTENS is being used to the point that a discernable muscle twitch is present. Such a response normally appears at 2-6Hz, which means 2.6 pulses per second. This level of stimulation has been shown to increase the body's release of endorphins, which, of course, creates a sense of wellbeing and dramatic pain relief.

This form of low-frequency, high-intensity stimulation tends to be more uncomfortable than conventional TENS therapy, and is often only tolerable in twenty- to thirty-minute sessions. However, the resulting pain relief is much longer lasting than that achieved via conventional TENS.

Safety Issues When Using TENS

In general, transcutaneous electrical nerve stimulation is well tolerated, although research is still ongoing. One must, however, exercise caution and never turn the TENS pulse generator up too high as this will likely cause over-stimulation and worsen the pain rather than relieve it.

The most prevalent complaint is minor skin irritation at the site of the electrode patches, but patients should be aware that electrical burns can occur when this method of passive pain relief therapy is misused.

TENS electrodes should never be placed on or near the eyes or in the mouth. Neither should they ever be placed on the temples or on the front of the neck. Broken or irritated skin should be avoided as well. People who suffer from decreased sensation or areas of numbness should use TENS with great caution.

Additionally, TENS should not be used on people who have implanted medical devices such as pacemakers, cardiac defibrillators or infusion pumps, as electric shock may occur or the devices may seriously malfunction.

Seizures have been occasionally reported as the result of TENS therapy. Therefore, it should be used very cautiously on people with seizure disorders such as epilepsy.

TENS and Back Pain

TENS is used to treat a wide variety of pain-producing medical conditions, including back pain, chronic pain, myofascial pain, and soft tissue injuries. Although studies as to its effectiveness are ongoing, TENS has enjoyed a healthy success rate.

As with other passive therapies, however, transcutaneous electrical nerve stimulation is most effective when teamed with other more active treatments such as chiropractic manipulation and specific exercise regimens.

Spinal Traction — Pulling Your Spine to Good Health?

Spinal traction boasts a long history in the treatment of various spinal maladies, including degenerative disk disease, joint dysfunction, and herniated or bulging disks. Although a number of traction techniques exist, the primary approach remains constant.

At a very basic level, spinal traction involves applying force to stabilize or change the positioning of damaged portions of the spine.

It is incredibly important to understand that spinal traction is only effective when it is part of a total treatment regimen, which must include other forms of treatment such as chiropractic manipulation or physical therapy. Without these more active treatment modalities, spinal traction has little if any chance of providing long-term benefit.

Looking Back at Spinal Traction's History

In the late 18th century, spinal traction achieved moderate recognition as a therapeutic option for the treatment of scoliosis and spinal deformity. It was also used in managing the ravaging symptoms of rickets and in the treatment of back pain.

Some physicians in the 19th century tried without success to utilize spinal traction as a means of treating a number of neurological disorders, including Parkinson's disease.

By the late 20th century, however, spinal traction became widely accepted as an appropriate treatment approach in the management of spinal trauma and pain.

In the early days of spinal traction, the methods of application frequently resulted in serious damage to the skin of the chin and neck, including severe pressure sores. These methods involved the application of various combinations of straps and harnesses to the head. This headgear was then connected to the weighted mechanism, which applied the actual traction force. The long-term use of this type of traction equipment was notorious for causing such excruciatingly painful skin damage.

Modern Uses for Spinal Traction

Today, the most commonly recognized use of spinal traction is for the management of cervical (neck) spine instability. This instability is caused by damage to the spinal column of the neck, and can be the result of either trauma or disease.

When such an instability occurs, the fragile vertebrae of the neck can shift or compress due to a misalignment, resulting in additional neurological (nerve) damage within the spinal column. The application of spinal traction can actually realign such a cervical spine dislocation and serves to stabilize the damaged spinal column.

Another interesting use of spinal traction addresses the symptoms associated with cervical radiculopathy. Put simply, the condition of cervical radiculopathy involves pain, numbness, tingling, and weakness in the arms and legs caused by a problem located in the spinal nerve roots located in the neck. Typically, this condition is caused by a spinal disk herniation.

Literally every disk in the spine can experience herniation, but the two most commonly affected areas are the neck and the lower back. When the herniation takes place in the neck, it is referred to as a cervical disk herniation, and when it occurs in the lower back, it is called a lumbar disk herniation.

An interesting side note is that lumbar disc herniation is much more common than cervical disk herniation, the former occurring fifteen times more often than the latter.

What Spinal Traction Does and How It Works

Modern spinal traction is based upon the application of an upward force to the skull while the rest of the body is held stationary. This upward force can be achieved either manually or mechanically. The objective is to stretch tight spinal muscles, relieve pinched nerves, and to change the position of damaged, misaligned, or compressed spinal vertebrae.

In the early 1980s, an exciting advance in mechanical spinal traction was introduced. Known as the Gardner-Wells tongs, this new device quickly replaced the more hazardous skull tongs previously associated with traction. The U-shaped Gardner-Wells tongs effectively control pressure at the sites of pin attachment to the skull, significantly decreasing the risk of pin penetration and the resulting skull damage. This device is commonly used when the traction treatment plan is short-term.

Another commonly used spinal traction device is the halo vest. This approach attaches a "halo," which is a piece of equipment that encircles and is fixed to the head of a patient, to a vest-like device that is worn around the torso. This halo vest is lightweight yet rigid, and fits snugly around a patient's chest. The result provides the needed continuous stability to the spine of the neck while also allowing for increased comfort and mobility.

For patients who require long-term treatment, use of the halo vest is certainly preferable to the Gardner-Wells tongs.

Manual Versus Mechanical

Determining whether manual or mechanical application of spinal traction is most appropriate depends upon each patient's individual physical condition.

For example, if a patient suffers from cervical radiculopathy (remember, this is pain, numbness, tingling, or weakness caused by a nerve root problem in the spine of the neck), mechanical traction is a likely choice. In this type of scenario, force is applied to the patient's skull by way of a halo vest paired with seven to ten pounds of traction weights, and is applied for about one hour three times daily. This kind of mechanical traction sometimes involves simply hanging the weights over a door while the patient is seated in a chair.

Manual spinal traction is often the better choice when the goal is to mobilize soft tissue or to treat impinged spinal facet joints. The force applied is gentle, stable, and controlled, utilizing hands, sand bags, and belts to achieve the desired spinal repositioning. The primary advantage in utilizing manual spinal traction is that range of motion can be easily incorporated into the spinal traction therapy.

Conventional Spinal Traction Is Not for Everyone

It is important to note that certain medical conditions, which impair or compromise the structural integrity of the spine, preclude the use of spinal traction as a treatment option. Primary examples of such conditions are osteoporosis, infection, presence of a tumor, or cervical rheumatoid arthritis. Additionally, pregnant patients as well as those with cardiovascular disease or a hernia are not good candidates for spinal traction.

When these health conditions are present, the use of spinal traction is potentially dangerous and should be avoided.

Spinal Decompression Boasts a High Rate of Success

Agonizing back pain is no respecter of persons. In fact, about 85% of the population will experience disabling back pain at least once in their lives. That averages out to approximately eight out of ten Americans. Sometimes the problem is aching or strained muscles. Other times, misaligned spinal vertebrae are the culprits.

But sometimes, the pain of spinal disk herniation, degenerative disk disease, arthritis, sciatica and other spinal conditions can hold you hostage, affecting every aspect of your day-to-day life. For these people, debilitating pain becomes an unwanted daily companion.

What Is a Herniated Disk and How Can Spinal Decompression Help?

The spinal disk is comprised of jelly-like tissue, and its function is to provide a cushion between each of the vertebrae in your spine. There is a protective outer band, called the annulus, and a soft middle section called the nucleus. Like a bubble on a tire, a herniated disk's nucleus bulges through a broken down or weak spot in the annulus, pressing up against the nearby nerves.

The result is nearly constant pain radiating down the back and into the legs, often causing reduced mobility and dysfunction.

In previous years, sufferers of herniated disks had but one option — a surgical procedure called a discectomy. However, with any surgery there are inherent risks such as excessive bleeding, nerve damage, and infection. And there is no guarantee that surgery will resolve the pain.

Clinical studies show that many times spinal decompression therapy is extremely effective in the treatment of herniated disks. As a matter of fact, the success rate is impressive. Equally exciting is the fact that another study has shown that the vast majority of herniated disk patients remain pain-free for four years after receiving spinal decompression therapy.

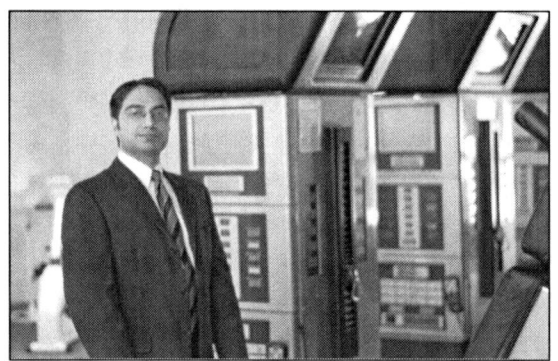

In the case of a herniated disk, spinal decompression therapy accomplishes two things. First, it increases the amount of space between the vertebrae, causing a negative pressure within the disk. The benefit of this negative pressure is that the bulging nucleus is drawn back inside the annulus where it belongs. Second, spinal decompression therapy increases the blood flow around and through the damaged disk, providing the oxygen and nutrients needed for the annulus to begin the process of healing the broken-down cartilage which caused the herniation.

What Exactly Is Spinal Decompression Therapy?

Spinal decompression therapy is a non-invasive method of treatment that has undergone the rigorous scrutiny and testing of the FDA and has received its 100% seal of approval. It is a highly effective method of treating not only herniated disks, but also chronic back pain and degenerative disk diseases.

Spinal decompression therapy is not conventional traction.

Conventional traction has been a standard form of back pain treatment for decades, but without any documented clinical efficacy. The problem with conventional traction is that it pulls both the muscles and the spine at the same time, often triggering very painful muscle spasms. This kind of generalized tension force does nothing to increase the height between the vertebrae.

On the other hand, spinal decompression therapy controls and isolates the amount of tension applied to a specific area of the spine. The result is pin-point accuracy in treating the exact spinal structures that are causing back pain. One might even offer the analogy that comparing conventional traction to spinal decompression therapy is like comparing a shotgun to a laser.

Spinal decompression therapy utilizes state-of-the-art computer-driven equipment. During such therapy, by cycling through gently applied pulling and relaxation phases, the pressure being exerted on spinal disks is carefully decreased while fluid exchange is enhanced. This fluid exchange is particularly vital to proper healing, since vertebral disks do not have blood vessels. This means that these disks require the diffusion of blood created by motion and decompression (a reduction in pressure) in order to receive the needed nutrients that enable and encourage healing.

Spinal decompression therapy has proven to be so effective that an article appearing in the Journal of Neurological Research stated: "We consider decompression therapy to be a primary treatment modality for low back pain associated with lumbar disk herniation at single or multiple levels, degenerative disk disease, facet arthropathy, and decreased spine mobility. We believe that post-surgical patients with persistent pain or 'failed back syndrome' should not be considered candidates for further surgery until a reasonable trial of decompression has been tried."

This highly respected medical publication also stated: "Decompression therapy addresses both primary and secondary causes of low back and referred leg pain. We submit that decompression therapy should be considered first before the patient undergoes a surgical procedure which permanently alters the anatomy and function of the affected lumbar spine segment."

Some Conditions Are Not Suitable for Spinal Decompression Therapy

Spinal decompression therapy is not an appropriate treatment for women who are pregnant. Additionally, patients who suffer severe osteoporosis, morbid obesity or severe nerve damage are not good candidates for spinal decompression.

If a patient has had a previous spinal surgery that included screws, metal plates or cages, spinal decompression therapy is not suitable. However, it can be performed with excellent results after bone fusion or non-fusion surgery.

Spinal Decompression Therapy Should Be Part of a Comprehensive Treatment Plan

As with any passive therapy, spinal decompression therapy achieves the best results when teamed with an active program of exercise and chiropractic manipulation to strengthen the spinal soft tissues. This kind of a well-rounded treatment program will restore muscle tone, increase range of motion, and stabilize the spinal vertebrae. It will also serve to correct any postural or muscle imbalances that may have been factors contributing to the low-back pain.

What Your Doctor Didn't Tell You about Medications

Literally millions of people in the United States alone take some sort of prescription drug every day. In fact, nearly half of all Americans take at least one prescription drug, and one in six takes three prescription drugs or more. Additionally, a growing number of people take over-the-counter medications and herbal products.

The result of combining an increased use of prescription drugs, over-the-counter medications and herbal supplements is an alarming potential for unexpected side effects as well as potentially hazardous interactions among these products.

Protect Yourself by Becoming an Informed Consumer

While prescription drugs have saved lives and improved the quality of life for millions, poisoning from prescription drugs has skyrocketed to become the Number Two cause of unintentional death in the United States. So the issue now becomes a matter of taking responsibility for our own bodies and our own health.

While your doctor is responsible for prescribing the right medication to treat your particular condition and your pharmacy is responsible for filling the prescription correctly, you should never be a passive bystander in matters of your health. Become proactive. Do research and ask questions. Learn what your prescriptions are supposed to do, how you should take them, and what their potential side effects might be. Educate yourself about the text on your prescription drug bottle. If there are any instructions or cautions that you do not understand or that cause you concern, discuss them with your physician or pharmacist.

Many pharmacies now feature prescription labeling that includes a brief physical description of the pill, capsule or liquid, such as "round, orange tablet scored across the center." Doctors are notorious for horribly indecipherable handwriting, and pharmacists are prone to the same human errors as the rest of us. So be sure that the physical description matches the contents of the bottle, and that the stated name and purpose of the drug matches what your doctor told you about the prescription before you take any medication.

Also, be sure your physician knows what medications you are currently taking, including any over-the-counter medicines or herbal supplements. This information is vital for your doctor to make an informed decision about a drug's potentially dangerous interaction with any of your other medications or supplements.

Drug Interactions Can Make Medications Less Effective or Even Dangerous

Basically, drug interactions fall into three categories. Any of these categories significantly increases the potential for unintended and unexpected interactions that can change the way a medication works.

First, let's discuss **drug-drug interactions.** This type of interaction can take place when two or more medications react to each other. For example, if you are taking an antihistamine for allergy problems, taking a sedative to help you sleep can make you extremely drowsy and slow your normal response time to a dangerous level. This becomes particularly hazardous if you are behind the wheel of a vehicle or operating machinery.

Another example of drug-drug interaction involves blood thinning medications such as Plavix® or Coumadin®. These prescription drugs help prevent blood clots in people who are at risk of heart attack or stroke. However, taking aspirin, naproxen, acetaminophen, or even the herb ginkgo biloba in combination with one of these blood-thinners can cause excessive bleeding.

The herbal supplement St. John's Wort is a popular natural treatment for mood swings and depression. However, it can have disastrous interactions with prescription and over-the-counter drugs alike. It can reduce the effectiveness of prescription drugs taken for the treatment of heart disease, depression, seizures, HIV, and certain types of cancer.

Next, **drug-beverage** or **food interactions** should be taken into consideration. The obvious example is taking a medication with alcohol. This combination can cause a myriad of dangerous, even lethal reactions.

Third on our list of basic drug interactions is **drug-health condition**. Certain medical conditions simply do not play well with specific types of medications. For example, nasal decongestants can perilously increase blood pressure when taken with prescription medications designed to treat high blood pressure.

Be Aware of Dangerous Side Effects

In 1999, Vioxx® was touted as the next miracle drug for pain relief. Doctors wrote over two million prescriptions to their patients who were suffering from arthritis and other painful joint disorders before it was disclosed that the use of Vioxx® increased the risk of heart attack and stroke by a shocking 50%. Subsequently, the FDA has estimated that this prescription drug may have caused up to 140,000 cases of serious heart disease since it was first introduced to the market.

Celebrex® is another popular arthritis medication that appears to more than double the risk of heart attack and other associated cardiovascular conditions.

Cholesterol-lowering drugs such as Crestor® have flooded the market as heart disease continues to reach an all-time high. However, many of these prescription medications designed to improve health actually cause extremely serious side effects. For example, Crestor® has been shown to cause kidney failure and muscle damage in an alarming number of consumers.

OxyContin® was approved by the FDA as a long-lasting, timed-released pain medication developed to manage moderate to severe pain. Typically, patients suffering from cancer, musculoskeletal conditions, and painful forms of paralysis were prescribed this medication. However, it was soon discovered that if these tablets were broken, chewed or crushed, a potentially fatal dose of medication was released into the bloodstream. OxyContin® has also earned a reputation as being even more addictive than heroin.

Ortho Evra® is a very popular contraceptive patch that has terrifying potential side effects. These side effects include blood clots, heart attack, stroke, and breast cancer.

And, of course, there is the hormone replacement therapy debacle. For years and years, doctors have prescribed drugs such as Prempro® to control the discomforts of menopause. Only in the last few years has it come to light that such prescription drugs significantly increase the risk of breast cancer, stroke, heart disease, and pulmonary embolism. In fact, the Women's Health Initiative determined that the risks associated with hormone replacement therapy vastly outweighed any potential benefits, and urged women to stop taking these drugs immediately.

Coping with Potential Side Effects

Most prescription drugs, as well as many over-the-counter medications, clearly list the known possible side effects of taking such a drug. Be sure to always read these potential side effects carefully. If you know what to expect and understand that any minor discomfort or inconvenience is only temporary, it is much less stressful and easier to deal with.

Here are some common medication side effects as well as suggestions on how to cope with them.

- ❖ **Diarrhea**   Drink plenty of water to replace the fluids lost through diarrhea. Do not take any diarrhea medications, even the over-the-counter ones. If this problem continues more than three days, you should call your doctor.

- ❖ **Constipation**   Be sure to drink at least ten glasses of water every day. Also increase the amount of fiber in your diet (carrots, apples and broccoli are great sources of fiber). Exercise is another good way to help relieve constipation.

- ❖ **Drowsiness or dizziness**   Do not drive or operate machinery. Also, check with your physician to see if you can take the medication at bedtime to help reduce these side effects. Also, when you stand, contract and relax your leg muscles for a few seconds before rising, then get up slowly.

- ❖ **Photosensitivity**   This side effect is extremely common with antibiotic medications and can cause you to suffer painfully severe sunburn in a matter of minutes. Apply sunscreen before you go outside, wear long-sleeved shirts and do not stay in the sunlight too long. Also, be sure to wear a hat to cover your scalp.

- ❖ **Nausea**   Take the medication with food or milk, and never on an empty stomach.

- ❖ **Itching**   Try taking warm (not hot) baths or showers fairly often. If a rash appears in conjunction with itching, you may be having an allergic reaction. If this occurs, be sure to contact your doctor.

- ❖ **Insomnia**   Ask your physician if you can take the medication earlier in the day. Also, avoid caffeine in the afternoon and evening.

- ❖ **Dry mouth**   Try sucking on sugarless hard candy or ice chips. Sugarless chewing gum also helps increase saliva.

- ❖ **Fluid retention**   Avoid highly salted foods and use a salt substitute to season your meals. Also, avoid drinking carbonated drinks such as colas. When seated, elevate your legs to above your heart. If you continue retaining fluid and gain more than three pounds in a week's time, you should talk to your doctor.

By educating yourself about medications, both prescription and over-the-counter, as well as having an open dialogue with your doctor, you can protect your health while also realizing maximum benefit from medications.

Managing Back Pain with Medication:
The Pros and Cons of Pain-killing Drugs

Basically, pharmaceuticals designed to help treat back pain come in two varieties. First, there are over-the-counter medications, also referred to as OTCs. The other form of pain management pharmaceuticals fall into the category of prescription drugs.

The drugs within these two varieties come in a number of shapes, sizes, and strengths. They also each come with specific risks, potential side effects, and interaction dangers.

Over-The-Counter Medications

Some of the more common over-the-counter, or OTC, pain relief medications include:

Naproxen sodium, which is marketed under the trade names of Aleve®, Anaprox®, Naprosyn®, Synflex® and Naprogesic®, is a non-steroidal anti-inflammatory drug (NSAID). Naproxen sodium is most often used to reduce fever, inflammation, and mild pain. It is generally effective when taken for conditions such as arthritis, gout, tendonitis, bursitis and injuries such as fractures.

The downside of naproxen sodium is that it can cause bleeding in the stomach and intestines. While rarely fatal, this side effect can occur without warning. However, the long-term use of this medication, when combined with the presence of heart disease, has been known to cause blood clots to form, resulting in heart attack and stroke.

Acetaminophen, whose common brand names include Tylenol® and Panadol®, is a common analgesic (painkiller) used to relieve fever, headaches, and minor aches and pains. It is a major ingredient in a number of cold and influenza medications, as well as several prescription pain medications.

While acetaminophen does not wreak the havoc on the stomach and intestines that naproxen sodium is known for, it can cause serious, irreversible liver damage when the recommended dosage is exceeded.

Ibuprofen is another non-steroidal anti-inflammatory drug. Its common brand names include Advil®, Motrin® and Nuprin®. Ibuprofen is commonly used to relieve the symptoms of arthritis, fever, and mild to moderate pain, particularly when inflammation is present. This NSAID is generally considered milder on the stomach than naproxen sodium, but only in daily dosages of less than 1,200mg.

Some of the common side effects of ibuprofen are nausea, gastrointestinal bleeding ulcers, diarrhea, dizziness, headache, and increased liver enzymes. It can also cause hypertension. In large doses, ibuprofen can cause kidney failure and even heart failure.

Prescription Pain Medication

When OTC pain relief medications prove to be simply not strong enough to provide adequate pain management, prescription pain medications become the next step in seeking pain relief. Here is a short list of the more commonly prescribed medications for back pain relief.

Cyclobenzaprine hydrochloride, which is marketed under the brand name of Flexeril®, is a skeletal muscle relaxant that relieves acute muscle spasms resulting from injuries such as sprains, strains, or pulls. Although cyclobenzaprine hydrochloride relieves the pain of strains and sprains, it is not useful for other types of pain.

One side effect of cyclobenzaprine hydrochloride is dry mouth. Sucking a hard candy, chewing gum, or melting ice chips in your mouth can provide temporary relief. The only other known side effect of this drug is occasional dizziness.

Metaxalone, whose common brand name is Skelaxin®, is another commonly pre-scribed muscle relaxant. This medication is used to reduce muscle pain and spasms typically associated with strains, sprains, or other muscle injuries.

Some of the more common side effects associated with metaxalone can include stomach upset, nausea, headache, dizziness, and dry mouth. Occasionally, more severe allergic reactions to this drug can occur. Symptoms of such an allergic reaction are itch-ing, swelling, difficulty breathing, and unexplained rash.

Oxycodone hydrochloride, marketed under the name of OxyContin®, is a highly addictive narcotic painkiller. OxyContin® is a controlled-release form of oxycodone prescribed to treat chronic pain. When used properly, OxyContin® can provide pain relief for up to twelve hours.

Oxycodone is among the most effective pain relievers available, providing up to four times the relief of other analgesics. Unlike other pain relief drugs such as aspirin or acetaminophen which have a threshold to their effectiveness, oxycodone has an increasing analgesic effect. Which means that the more you take, the better you feel.

Common side effects are constipation, nausea, sedation, dizziness, vomiting, head-ache, dry mouth, sweating, and weakness. The most serious risk associated with oxycodone is respiratory depression. Taking a large single dose of a narcotic such as oxycodone can cause severe respiratory depression leading to death.

Another form of oxycodone hydrochloride is Percocet®. Unlike OxyContin™, the formulation of Percocet™ includes acetaminophen. This narcotic is routinely prescribed for post-operative pain control as well as for the treatment of moderate to severe chronic pain.

In addition to the previously listed oxycodone side effects and risks, the presence of acetaminophen in the drug presents a risk of dangerous liver damage and gastro-intestinal distress.

Hydrocodone and acetaminophen, marketed under the brand Vicodin®, is a Schedule III narcotic, which means that it has a high psychological dependence and low-to-medium physical addiction. Vicodin® is most commonly prescribed for patients experiencing surgical-related pain or other intense pain.

Side effects of Vicodin® include hyperventilation, seizures, severe weakness and fatigue, clammy skin, unexplained bleeding, and unconsciousness. Other known side effects are jaundice, hearing loss, and a decreased sex drive. This narcotic formulation also has depressant effects on the central nervous system and, since it contains acet-aminophen, the danger of liver damage is also present.

Painkiller Addiction

While NSAIDs are not narcotic and are, therefore, non-addictive, narcotic pharmaceu-ticals such as oxycodone and hydrocodone are highly addictive.

Addiction to pain relief medications can be defined as the compulsive use of a substance. This behavior is characterized by a loss of control over yourself and your life. The goal of obtaining more and more of a specific drug takes precedence over your job, your family, and even your health.

One of the warning signs of drug addiction is a change in personality, such as a shift in energy, mood or focus. Other red flags are social withdrawal, blackouts or forgetful-ness, unusual neglect of responsibilities, and defensiveness about taking the drug.

Drug Tolerance

Over time, it is quite common for someone taking prescription medications to develop a tolerance to the effects of the medication's prescribed dosage. The drug of choice just no longer provides the same pain relief or "high" that it did initially, so a progressively larger dosage is needed to achieve the desired effect.

In addicted individuals, this resulting pattern of uncontrolled escalation of doses oftentimes leads to drug overdose.

Physical Dependence on Painkillers

When one is physically dependent upon addictive pain relieving drugs, withdrawal symptoms manifest during abstinence.

Although being addicted to a narcotic drug implies drug dependence, it is possible to be dependent without being addicted. For example, people who regularly take pharmaceuticals to treat a disease or health disorder may experience an improvement in their condition, even though the drug interferes with their ability to function. These people are considered dependent upon a particular drug, but not addicted to it.

Both prescription and over-the-counter medications can be safe when taken according to label directions or a doctor's instructions. However, they can also be extremely dangerous and even life-threatening. Use all drugs with caution and only for as long as they are absolutely necessary, and never, ever exceed the recommended dosages.

Anti-Inflammatory Pain Medications: What Your Choices Are and How They Affect Your Body

The most commonly used medications to relieve pain, inflammation, and fever are non-steroidal anti-inflammatory drugs, often referred to simply as NSAIDs. For sufferers of back pain, arthritis, bursitis, tendonitis, and generalized joint pain, NSAIDs can provide a fresh breath of relief, but can also pose significant risks to your health.

NSAIDs come in two varieties – over-the-counter and prescription.

You have probably used several of the most common over-the-counter without giving much thought to what they are or how they work. Popular over-the-counter NSAID brand names include Motrin® and Advil®, which contain ibuprofen. Other popular choices are Aleve® and Naprosyn®, which contain naproxen sodium. Even the common aspirin is a non-steroidal anti-inflammatory drug.

When prescription NSAIDs are required for a stronger form of relief, your doctor might prescribe Toradol®, Celebrex®, DayPro® or Relafen®.

For example, if you suffer from rheumatoid arthritis, you might receive a prescription for a higher dosage of NSAIDs as this type of health condition usually causes severe swelling, redness, and joint stiffness. For other maladies such as osteoarthritis or acute muscle injuries, lower doses of a prescription NSAID are often effective since there is usually less joint swelling or redness.

How NSAIDs Work

Non-steroidal anti-inflammatory medications block the effect of an enzyme called cyclooxygenase. Now don't let this dry, medical-sounding name dull your interest because understanding how NSAIDs work is not only interesting, it can also be vital to protecting your health.

Cyclooxygenase is essential in the production of prostaglandins, a hormone-like enzyme that occurs naturally in your body. Prostaglandins are the culprits that cause the pain, fever and swelling of arthritis, bursitis, and tendonitis, just to name a few. It would seem obvious that blocking their effect would be a good thing.

However, prostaglandins do something else as well. Specifically, one particular variety of prostaglandin is responsible for lining the stomach with a protective fluid called gastric mucosa.

So, by blocking cyclooxygenase, NSAIDs also interfere with the hormone that helps protect your stomach from ulcers. This can lead to a cascade of incredibly serious health risks.

Dangerous NSAID-related Adverse Effects

Serious health problems can develop without warning as a result of taking non-steroidal anti-inflammatory medications.

As just mentioned, NSAIDs are known to frequently cause stomach ulcers. And sometimes, these stomach ulcers worsen to the point that they begin to bleed. In far too many cases, the bleeding becomes severe enough that hospitalization becomes necessary and can even result in death.

The variables in determining when, and if, bleeding ulcers become life-threatening appear to be the type of drug, the dosage, the duration of exposure, and existing patient characteristics.

For example, if someone has a history of stomach ulcers or if they are taking a blood-thinner like Warfarin or Coumadin due to heart or stroke risk, NSAIDs would be an extremely poor choice. Also, patients over the age of 60 are more prone to dangerous stomach ulceration, as are those who smoke or drink alcohol.

So, how big is the problem of gastrointestinal adverse effects? According to a major study, there are over 100,000 NSAID-related hospital admissions every year in the United States alone.

Even more shocking, more than 16,500 deaths each year are attributed to the adverse effects of NSAIDs.

The United Kingdom comes in second behind the U.S. with 12,000 annual NSAID-related hospital admissions and 2,600 NSAID-related deaths.

Traditional NSAIDs Versus COX-2 Inhibitors

While traditional NSAIDs block the production of *all* prostaglandins, the problem is that there are several varieties of this hormone. Some varieties result in painful inflammation, and others line the stomach with protective liquid. The prostaglandins that cause inflammation are COX-2 enzymes, and the prostaglandins that help protect the stomach are COX-1 enzymes.

So the problem becomes how to block one enzyme without shutting down the other.

Enter the new generation of NSAIDs called COX-2 inhibitors. These medications relieve pain and inflammation just as effectively as traditional NSAIDs, but with an interesting twist. They target inflammation-causing COX-2 enzymes only, while allowing beneficial COX-1 enzymes to do their work unimpeded.

Thus, COX-2 inhibitors help relieve pain and inflammation with the added benefit of protecting your stomach from ulcers and bleeding. Additionally, COX-2 inhibitors do not appear to significantly impede blood clotting, making it a much safer choice for patients who take blood thinning drugs or who are preparing for surgery.

Currently, Celebrex® is the only prescription COX-2 inhibitor on the market. Vioxx® and Bextra®, also COX-2 inhibitors, were removed from the market after FDA testing revealed an alarming increase in heart attack and stroke associated with these medications.

NSAID Usage

There is no way to completely bullet-proof yourself against the side effects of any drug you may be taking, but there are steps you can take to minimize the risks associated with non-steroidal anti-inflammatory medications.

For example, use any NSAID, whether over-the-counter or prescription, with caution. Be sure to follow directions very carefully. Over-the-counter NSAIDSs are designed for short-term use, so if you need to take an OTC NSAID for more than two weeks, talk to your physician. If the NSAID is a prescription medication, take it only for the amount of time that your doctor has recommended.

Take NSAIDs with food and a full glass of water to minimize the risk of stomach irritation. If you experience stomach distress that lasts for more than a few days, contact your physician.

If you miss a dose of NSAIDs, do not ever take a double dose. If it nearly time for your next dose, simply skip the missed dose and go back to your regular medication schedule.

Be sure to ask your doctor before taking any vitamin/mineral supplements or homeopathic compounds. Like any other over-the-counter or prescription medication, NSAIDs can have dangerous interactions with other health products or medications.

Also, if you need to take an additional over-the-counter pain reliever, use an acetaminophen product such as Tylenol® instead of ibuprofen. This is especially important to remember if you have an ulcer or are at a high risk of developing stomach ulcers.

If you are on a daily aspirin regimen, use coated aspirin to help prevent the medication from irritating your stomach.

Consider asking your doctor about taking a prescription acid blocker if you are at an increased risk of ulcers.

NSAID Side Effects

The most common side-effect complaints regarding NSAID treatment are mild nausea, indigestion, and heartburn. These can usually be avoided by taking the medication with food and plenty of water.

Other minor side effects can include mild diarrhea, headache, lightheadedness, or drowsiness. You might also experience a slight ringing in the ears or even a mild rash. Should you experience any of these side effects, talk to your doctor. There may be alternative treatments that will not be quite so bothersome, yet still be effective in the relief of your pain and inflammation.

Severe side effects can occur with NSAID use, including the gastrointestinal problems discussed earlier, as well as kidney failure and worsening of pre-existing congestive heart failure. Should you experience any of the following symptoms, you should stop taking the NSAID and contact your doctor immediately.

* Severe nausea, heartburn or abdominal pain

* Bloody or black, tarry stools

* Vomiting blood or tissue

* Severe bruising

* Shortness of breath or difficulty breathing

* Elevated blood pressure

* Tightness in the chest or chest pain

* Convulsions or seizures

- ❖ Unexplained weight gain
- ❖ Sudden decrease in urinary output

All About Muscle Relaxant Medications: What They Are, How They Work and What To Watch Out For

After any type of soft tissue injury, muscles can tend to tighten up and spasm. This is actually a protective reaction on the part of your musculature, but it can certainly result in pain and limited range of motion.

If you have ever suffered a muscle strain, sprain, or other soft tissue injury, your doctor may have prescribed a muscle relaxant to help relieve the pain, stiffness, and discomfort. Like all medications, muscle relaxants should be taken with caution and only after you have researched the possible adverse side effects.

It is important to realize that muscle relaxant medications will not heal a muscle injury. Nor can they take the place of rest, careful exercise, and other therapy your doctor may recommend, such as chiropractic manipulation.

A word of caution is in order. While taking a muscle relaxant drug can make you feel better, your body is still going through the process of healing. So use caution and common sense when it comes to physical exertion and heavy lifting in order to avoid worsening your injury.

How Muscle Relaxants Work

Muscle relaxant medications do not actually work directly on skeletal muscles. Rather, they work in the brain and central nervous system, and actually relax your entire body instead of specific musculature. These medications appear to be much more effective in the relief of muscle pain or spasms than either acetaminophen or aspirin.

These pain relief medications may be administered orally or the medication may be injected directly into the spinal canal, depending upon which drug is prescribed. However, all drugs in the muscle relaxant class can cause sedation, and when administered into the spinal canal, severe central nervous system depression can occur. This is a very dangerous reaction that can result in cardiovascular collapse and even respiratory failure.

The presence of medical problems other than your current muscle sprain, strain, or other soft tissue injury can affect the use of a skeletal muscle relaxant. Be sure to tell your doctor if you have any known allergies, kidney disease, liver disease, blood disorders, epilepsy, or porphyria. If you are a female, it is also important to let your doctor know if you are pregnant or a nursing mom.

Four Most Commonly Prescribed Muscle Relaxants

Carisoprodol, marketed under the brand names of Soma®, Rela®, and Venadom®, is a muscle relaxer that works by blocking pain sensations between the nerves and the brain.

Often prescribed to manage the pain of soft tissue injuries and other musculoskeletal conditions, carisoprodol may be habit-forming. This type of muscle relaxant medication can impair your ability to think clearly, and may slow your normal reactions. So exercise caution should you need to drive or do anything that requires you to be awake and alert. Also avoid drinking alcohol, as it can increase any drowsiness and dizziness caused by this medication.

Metaxalone, sold under the brand name of Skelaxin®, has been shown to produce medically significant results in patients with muscle spasm or decreased flexibility. This medication is meant to be used only in acute situations and only for a short period of time, typically no more than three weeks. Although metaxalone appears to function as a sedative, it is not completely known how it actually works.

Like carisoprodol, metaxalone does not directly relax skeletal muscles. Instead, it addresses pain via the central nervous system, providing an "all over" sense of relaxation.

This medication can enhance the effects of alcohol, barbiturates, and other central nervous system depressants. Additionally, metaxalone can cause drowsiness.

An important note about metaxalone to diabetics — this medication has been known to cause false blood sugar test results. Monitor your glucose levels very carefully. If you notice an unusually sharp increase in sugar levels, be sure to check with your doctor immediately.

Cyclobenzaprine, marketed as Flexeril®, can be used safely for longer periods of time than either carisoprodol or metaxalone. Although cyclobenzaprine relieves the pain of strains and sprains, it has not proven to be useful for other types of pain.

While it is not an antidepressant, its chemical structure is very similar to several antidepressant medications. Therefore, cyclobenzaprine should not be taken if you are taking an MAO (monoamine oxidase) inhibitor antidepressant drug or if you have taken such an MAO inhibitor within two weeks prior to cyclobenzaprine being prescribed to you.

Additionally, cyclobenzaprine should be avoided if you have been diagnosed with congestive heart failure, if you suffer from an irregular heartbeat, or if you have recently experienced a heart attack.

Diazepam, also known as Valium®, is an effective muscle relaxant and pain reliever when low back pain or muscle spasms are present. In addition to addressing muscle spasms and pain, diazepam is used to relieve anxiety, nervousness and tension associated with anxiety disorders.

This medication is highly habit-forming and is known to dramatically change sleep cycles. Therefore, the use of diazepam should be limited to no more than one or two weeks. Also, diazepam is a known depressant and can actually worsen any symptoms of depression associated with chronic back pain.

Side Effects, from Common to Rare

Some minor side effects may occur as your body adjusts to the type of muscle relaxant medication you are taking and generally do not require the attention of your doctor. These can include blurred or double-vision, dizziness, and lightheadedness.

Somewhat less common side effects can include a fast heartbeat, fainting, skin rash, shortness of breath or difficulty breathing, stuffy nose, bloodshot eyes, depression, confusion, constipation, diarrhea, nervousness, hiccups, headache, heartburn, and stomach cramps.

Serious side effects, although rare, should be reported immediately to your physician. Side effects that should raise a red flag of alarm include blood in your urine, bloody or black stools, seizures, painful or sharply decreased urination, swollen or painful glands, vomiting blood or tissue, jaundice, and unusual bruising or bleeding.

Virtually every pharmaceutical has the potential for side effects, whether it is over-the-counter or prescription. Some side effects can be simply bothersome, but others can seriously, even fatally, impact your health and wellbeing. For this reason, you should weigh both the benefits and the possible hazards of any medication prior to taking it — including muscle relaxant drugs.

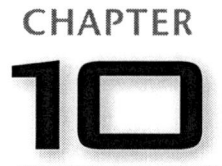
Invasive Conservative Treatments for Back Pain

Injections That Go Straight to The Source of Your Back Pain

Since conservative therapies do not always work, it is reassuring to know that a happy medium exists between medication and surgery. For the patient who has tried nearly every medication available, there are options. There are still conservative therapy options for the individual who has spent months or even years masking the pain rather than treating its source.

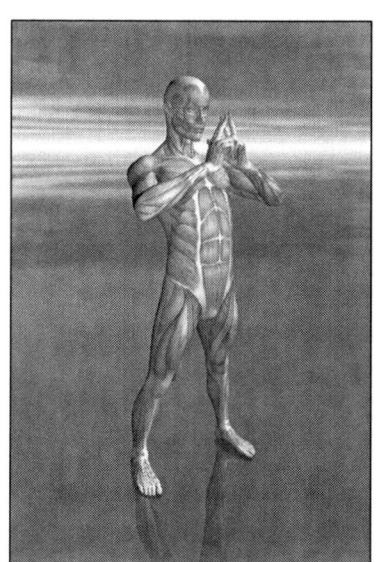

Active physical therapy is one of the few methods that treat the source of pain rather than covering it, but if weak muscles are not the true root of the back pain, it simply will not work. If this description sounds like you, it would be wise for you to research a few invasive conservative treatment options before agreeing to go under the knife. Many of these invasive conservative therapies are injections but there is truly a wide range of alternatives from which to choose.

Some of the most effective treatments are seldom heard of and virtually unknown to the common patient. For example, trigger point therapy has been dubbed an alternative treatment option in many respects. However, many physicians offer this service to patients suffering from back pain; thus, it is growing in popularity and quickly becoming a more traditional option for alleviating back pain.

Here is how it works:

Trigger Point Injections

Trigger points are sensitive areas of the muscle and are typically associated with palpable nodules, which are tense, knotted areas of a muscle. In many cases, they can be felt beneath the surface of the skin. Additionally, this type of therapy works best when muscles are damaged do to injury or repeated muscle strain. Moreover, trigger points affect not only that particular muscle but also nerves surrounding it.

During a therapy session, a small amount of local anesthetic is injected into the trigger point, which deactivates the irritated area. The anesthetic scrambles the signals that cause painful sensations in the nerves, leaving the area more relaxed.

Even if a patient is allergic to this form of medication, dry needle techniques can be used on trigger points. Dry needle techniques simply mean that the needles have no medication. Instead, the physician uses the needle as a tool to stimulate the muscle rather than a means of delivering medication. Though dry needling causes more soreness than regular trigger point injections, it is usually just as effective. Trigger point injections should only be used on one muscle per session and the patient should only receive three or less injections per trigger point.

This limitation helps protect the patient from scarring and other potential damage to the muscle. Also, trigger point injections should be reserved for patients who have not responded to four or more weeks of passive therapy such as medication.

In most cases, when an individual experiences muscle strain, a short rest period, pain management therapy (medication, hot and cold therapies, etc.), and slow reintroduction of normal daily activities allow the patient enough time to heal from the injury. Thus, more invasive therapies such as trigger point injections are more suitable for patients not affected by more passive treatment options.

Most physicians prescribe an active physical program to be implemented along with the injections. Regular exercise facilitates flexibility, adds strength, and conditions the muscles. Most importantly, exercise prevents re-injury of the muscles because they become stronger. More strength means less fatigue and fewer opportunities for muscle strain.

Prolotherapy

Like trigger point therapy, this type of treatment is not well-known. Still, it has proven to be effective in providing relief for patients experiencing back pain. While trigger point therapy is geared more toward alleviating pain from sore muscles, prolotherapy involves pain in the joints.

Like trigger point therapy, prolotherapy involves an injection that is basically placed directly into the irritated area; thus, prolotherapy is dispensed through an injection in or near a sore joint. While the ingredients in a given solution will vary depending upon the condition being treated, prolotherapy injections work by reducing inflammation. Once inflammation decreases, blood circulation increases. This delivers more oxygen and nutrients to the area. Additionally, it cleanses the area of irritating toxins that only contribute to pain and inflammation.

Moreover, proponents of prolotherapy theorize that improved circulation allows new cells to ligaments, tendons, and surrounding tissues which in turn leads to healthier joints.

Also, prolotherapy is most often used to treat areas of the spine which are subject to ligament injuries. The components, location, quantity, and intervals of each injection will vary according to the patient's condition. Of course, practitioners usually recommend stretching exercises to aid in healthy tissue production, spinal manipulation to maintain mobility, or physical therapy to strengthen and condition muscles.

Many Other Invasive Conservative Treatments Offered

Trigger point injections and prolotherapy provide only a couple of examples among the variety of invasive conservative treatment options. What is more, the best way to make a healthy, informed decision is to consult a physician. Depending on the source of your back pain, he will prescribe the treatment that suits your needs best. Of course, doing your own preliminary research helps give you a better understanding of what to expect; thus, you may know well before your physician whether you are responding to a recommended therapy.

When Back Pain Gets on Your Nerves

There are numerous conditions that trigger back pain. The cause may be something as simple as sleeping in the wrong position, poor posture, or even a sports injury. It might be a result of repetitive lifting or bending that eventually takes its toll on muscles, leaving them fatigued or strained.

While muscle strain is a very common cause of back pain, it is not the only one. Rather, many people encounter back pain because of pressure or damage to nerves. In fact, these nerves are most often located along the spine and near the spinal cord. They are highly sensitive and when they are irritated, they can make even the simplest daily activities agonizing.

Since the pain seems so overwhelming, many people who are struggling with this type of back pain assume they are in need of surgery. No matter how intense the pain may be, there are alternatives to surgery. These methods are more invasive that traditional conservative treatment options, but patients are best served when they exhaust all options before seriously considering surgery.

Selective Nerve Root Block (SNRB)

When a nerve root is constricted, it causes pain and inflammation in the lower back and occasionally, in one or both legs. While practitioners typically use an MRI to diagnose this condition, it does not always shed light on which nerve is causing the irritation. Because of its diagnostic properties, a selective nerve root block is particularly useful in situations such as this. SNRB can is also effective as treatment for a far lateral disc herniation.

This is how an SNRB works. First, a solution consisting of a steroid (to act as an anti-inflammatory) and lidocaine (to act as a numbing agent) is injected into the area between the vertebrae. Of course, many patients are especially wary of needles being placed anywhere near the spine. With this being such a delicate area, this fear is certainly understandable.

You can take comfort in the fact that nerve root blocks are done under the supervision of a live X-ray, which helps the practitioner make certain the injection takes place in the correct location. If you experience pain relief after the SNRB, it is safe to assume that the injected nerve root was in fact the source of your discomfort and that this form of treatment is proving itself effective.

If back pain recurs, it may be possible to repeat this form of therapy. Most physicians will do a nerve root block up to three times per year. Lastly, it is important to keep in mind that nerve root blocks are followed by a short period of increased leg pain in some patients.

Facet Joint Block

Facet joints are paired along the spine; additionally, they have opposing cartilage surfaces and share a surrounding capsule. Pain in this area usually begins with a twisting injury, but it is also caused by cartilage degeneration found in elderly patients.

Facet joint block injections offer relief for patients experiencing this type of back pain. They work similarly to selective nerve root block injections. They have diagnostic capabilities and they consist of a steroid and lidocaine combination.

Like the selective nerve root block, facet joint injections are guided by a live X-ray. The best way to determine the effectiveness of this treatment is to see whether it is successful in alleviating back pain. If back pain returns, facet joint blocks may be repeated up to three times a year.

Radiofrequency Radioablation

Nerve blocks can be effective for weeks or even months of relief but, unfortunately, the pain resumes for some patients. In cases such as these, radiofrequency radioablation may provide the most effective pain relief. Though this treatment option is minimally invasive, requiring only an injection, it is also fairly drastic.

Many consider it drastic because it permanently deadens the nerve. Additionally, remember that nerves are in place for a specific purpose, and that reason is to make you aware of abnormal conditions in the body. Deadening a nerve only causes it to go silent; therefore, this does not address the conditions that are placing unnecessary pressure on the nerve in the first place.

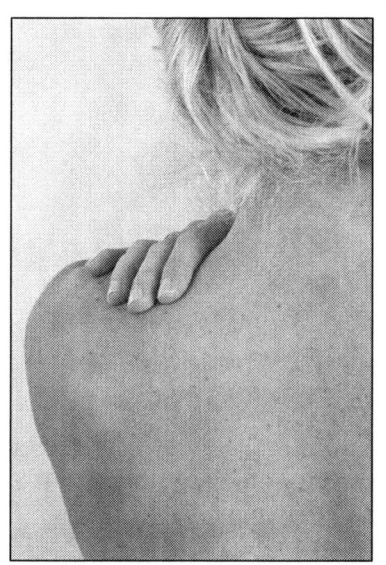

If other conservative therapies have failed in alleviating the pain, radiofrequency radioablation may be a method available, especially if it prevents you from undergoing spinal surgery, which is truly the most drastic treatment a patient could ever consider.

For back pain that goes beyond sore muscles and straight to sensitive nerves located along the spine, injections such as these are most often an effective form of treatment. When dealing with pressure on the nerves, going through treatment after treatment can be very frustrating.

It seems easy to throw your hands up and head to the operating room. However, holding out and trying as many conservative treatments as possible is truly worth the effort. After all, once surgery has been performed, there is no going back. Furthermore, the surgery itself can produce even more complications. For example, many patients do not recover well; they may even have scar tissue as a result of going through surgery.

The Epidural Space of The Spine: It May Lead to Pain Relief

With so many different back pain therapies offered to patients, it might be difficult to know which one may be the best one for you. Of course, this is why it is imperative to take the advice of a physician in addition to conducting your own research. Still, even those patients who stay extra busy investigating the many treatment opportunities may not know or completely understand how they work.

You do not have to be a physician or specialist to understand what is accessible and how it works. All that is necessary is a small amount of time and effort. Taking the time to make inquiries will prove to be well worth your efforts, especially if you are able to avoid going through an invasive procedure.

As you may have learned, an invasive procedure most often refers to a surgical procedure. More specifically, it requires an incision. Additionally, there are non-invasive methods that call for neither needle nor knife. Instead, they rely on conservative approaches such as massage or prescribed exercises. Somewhere in between very different approaches to treating back pain, invasive conservative therapies are available.

They usually do not involve any incisions. Rather, most of them are injections or use catheters. There are several different approaches to delivering pain relief to the affected area. Treatments that rely on injections or catheters often rely on the epidural space of the spine.

When most people think of an epidural, they think of a pregnant woman who receives an epidural to help manage her labor pain. However, there are various types of epidurals. Following are a couple of examples.

Epidural Steroid Injections (ESI)

ESIs are typically used to alleviate pain caused by stenosis, spondylolysis, herniated disc and irritated nerve roots. First of all, stenosis is characterized by narrowing of the spinal and root canal, which causes pain in the back and leg. This pain is more noticeable when walking.

Spondylolysis, on the other hand, is a condition in which a weak area or fracture is found between the upper and lower facets of the vertebrae. If the vertebrae shift forward, they may press against the nerve, triggering back pain. And finally, a herniated disc occurs when the jelly-like substance within the vertebral disc seeps out. This places pressure on the nearby nerves and, thus, causes back pain. Additionally, an ESI may be used to treat inflammation, particularly when it is brought on by a herniated disc.

This type of injection is administered around the dura, which is the sac surrounding the nerve roots. The dura contains cerebrospinal fluid, the liquid in which nerve roots are immersed. As with any procedure involving the spine, many patients do not know what to expect, which makes the process somewhat intimidating.

However, this treatment option is fairly straightforward. Within the first few minutes after receiving the injection, your legs may feel numb and heavy. This is from the local anesthetic and this effect will remain for several hours. Of course, after this initial time has passed, you will encounter some soreness for two or three days. After that, you will notice pain relief.

Because the ESI contains steroids, it has the capability to act as an anti-inflammatory. Not only does it provide pain relief, it offers freedom to a once stiffened, constricted area. In addition, improved circulation cleanses the area of accumulated toxins that cause pain.

Since ESIs are not always effective (over 50 percent of patients who receive an ESI experience pain relief as a result), they are only used as a last resort once you and your physician have determined that other conservative treatments are not right for you.

As with any medical treatment, there are some risks to those who receive an ESI. If the needle is placed too far, spinal headaches, infection, nerve damage, bleeding, and arachnoiditis can occur. Moreover, it can trigger weight gain and water retention in some patients as well as elevated blood sugar levels in diabetic patients.

Epidural Lysis of the Adhesions

When scar tissue forms around a nerve near the spinal cord, it restricts movement, causing inflammation. The tight and inflamed muscles causes back pain. This condition can be very frustrating, especially since it is most common among patients recovering from back surgery.

Still, it may also be the result of chronic inflammation of the nerve, which provides an example of why back pain should always be addressed. At any rate, lysis of adhesions provides the opportunity for pain relief. First, a local anesthetic is administered. Then, a spring-guided catheter is placed in the epidural space, directed by live X-ray. Once the catheter reaches the irritated nerve roots, the medication is distributed directly to the cause of the pain. Over the next few days, the medication begins to break down the adhesions, which also helps with inflammation. Furthermore, subsequent visits may be required in order to take care of all the adhesions causing the pain.

Pain Relief Has Become Portable

As technology continues to rapidly advance, treatment options for various medical conditions continue to provide better healing, better pain management and, fortunately, better quality of life for patients throughout the world. Most importantly, for those challenged by back pain, these advances translate to more and more options available and fewer incidences where surgery is the only option for pain relief.

Since surgery is not effective for many patients and can even lead to further complications, people look to conservative treatment options. They are utilizing passive and active therapies and exhausting their options before agreeing to allow physicians to perform surgery on their bodies.

Though this takes a great deal of time and effort, it often leads to pain relief that is long lasting or even permanent. Such is not always the case with surgery. Moreover, if they are willing, patients have the opportunity to make use of invasive conservative therapies. Of course, some are more invasive than others.

Implantable treatment methods, for example, often require a small incision and will be worn at all times. Both intrathecal drug delivery systems and spinal cord stimulators are examples of implantable therapies. If you prefer to manage pain with medication or are interested in exploring electrotherapy, one of these treatment options may be for you.

Intrathecal Drug Delivery

Like injection treatments, intrathecal drug delivery is designed to distribute medication directly to the irritated area causing back pain. The main feature of this treatment is that it uses a catheter and pump to transport medication. It works by administering medication through the intrathecal area surrounding the spinal cord.

The pump itself is surgically implanted below the skin of the abdomen; it is connected to a catheter with its subcutaneous path to the site at which medication is to be delivered. Before implementing this treatment method, the physician will execute a trial phase to determine whether a patient will respond well to the medication.

In some cases, the physician may opt to release medication to the intrathecal area of the spinal cord via injection rather than through a catheter. Or, the physician may decide to use a pump that is worn externally for a few days instead of a surgically implanted one. The most notable difference between an injection therapy and intrathecal drug delivery is that intrathecal drug delivery most often provides medication in smaller doses at a set rate. In contrast, patients who receive facet, epidural, or nerve block injections are typically given three or fewer injections per year.

Spinal Cord Stimulator (SCS)

This type of treatment is effective because it relies on electrical impulses to inhibit the brain's ability to detect pain. Like many other invasive conservative treatments, many patients are unaware of this option and do not understand how it works. Though it may seem intimidating to some patients, the process is actually very simple and only minimally invasive.

First, fine, pliable wires are placed through a needle going into the back near the spine. Then, a small incision is made to allow placement of the small programmable generator beneath the skin of the buttock or abdomen. Finally, this generator produces electrical currents that distract the brain from sensations of pain.

SCS is used to treat an assortment of conditions that cause chronic back pain. These include: arachnoiditis (inflammation of the meninges, the protective layers of the spine), causalgia (pain caused by peripheral nerve injury), failed back surgery syndrome (occurs when surgery is unsuccessful in providing pain relief for the back and/or extremities), peripheral neuropathy (pain in the legs caused by distant nerve endings that are dying) and reflex sympathetic dystrophy (also known as complex regional pain syndrome and is characterized by constant pain caused by this progressive nervous system disorder).

Since all patients respond to treatment differently, the intensity of electrical stimulation can be changed by the patient. The initial programming is done by a physician. Still, patients are given the chance to learn how to control the generator's output according to their needs. Additionally, there is more than one variety of spinal cord stimulation available.

Similar to the standard SCS, Peripheral Nerve Field Stimulation (PNFS) also uses pleasant electric currents to replace sensations of pain. The key difference here is that PNFS is located near the nerve as opposed to a less specific place in the lower back or abdomen.

Though invasive conservative therapies are far safer than surgery, they should still be considered with caution. Furthermore, they should be sought out only by those not responding to more conservative treatments such as chiropractic treatment, passive treatments, or physical therapy. Still, these methods may be unsuccessful in providing pain relief or inappropriate for the type of pain you are experiencing.

Invasive Therapies Prove Beneficial

People experiencing muscle pain often rely on heat to provide pain relief. Because heat causes blood vessels to dilate, it allows the irritated area to flush itself out. This removes built-up toxins that make existing pain even worse. When combined with cold therapy (ice), which constricts the vessels and reduces inflammation, it is especially effective.

However, when dealing with nerve pain, heat must be used in a very different way. Intradiscal electrothermal therapy (IDET) delivers heat using a catheter. While it is very beneficial in alleviating back pain, there is some risk to surrounding tissues, which can be damaged by the heat. Radiofrequency discal nucleoplasty provides very similar back pain relief without the higher temperatures. Of course, this helps keep surrounding tissues safe. Though both treatment methods target pain caused by irritated nerves, there are some key differences.

Intradiscal Electrothermal Therapy (IDET)

IDET therapy is very beneficial for those who have chronic back pain due to cracking of an intervertebral disc. Fractures in an intervertebral disc are most often caused by old age or by injury to this area. Moreover, the inner disc tissue may cause the disc to become herniated, which causes them to protrude into these cracks.

This triggers even more pain to the affected disc. Fortunately, IDET provides effective pain relief for those who experience discomfort from fractures or disc herniation. This treatment method is minimally invasive, requiring only a numbing injection and a catheter.

Here is how it works: First, with the assistance of a live X-ray, the physician inserts a needle into the disc. Next, she guides a catheter through the needle into the disc where it will gradually become warmer. Moreover, the heat contracts and thickens collagen in the disc's wall in addition to raising the temperature of the nerve endings.

The temperature increases to about 90 degrees Celsius and the treatment session lasts approximately 15 to 17 minutes. During this process, the thickened collagen fibers encourage the cracks to close. Moreover, heat also cauterizes the nerve endings. As the nerve endings become burned, they lose sensitivity, which helps to ensure pain relief. And lastly, the catheter is removed.

Patients are allowed to go home after only a short observation period. Over the next 12 to 16 weeks after the treatment, you should experience pain relief as disc wall fractures begin to close in addition to reduction of disc herniation and desensitization of nerves within the disc.

You may encounter some initial discomfort until several days after the procedure when the disc is no longer heated. Your physician may prescribe medication to help manage the pain until then. Additionally, most patients wear lumbar support for six to eight weeks after IDET, allowing the area to heal safely. Still, it is vital that you treat your spine with care as the healing process takes place. Your physician will provide guidelines on when and how to safely resume physical activity.

Radiofrequency Discal Nucleoplasty (Coblation Nucleoplasty)

This treatment method is very similar to IDET but it is more conducive to reducing a herniated disc than repairing the fissures. Therefore, patients are better served if they rely on this treatment option for alleviating sciatica-like pain. (This type of pain usually occurs in the lower back and leg.)

Like IDET, radiofrequency discal nucleoplasty is a short outpatient procedure, lasting approximately 30 to 60 minutes. It includes a high-frequency probe that emits a plasma field instead of heat. This plasma field breaks apart the molecular bonds in the collagen of the nucleus, essentially disintegrating it. At the conclusion of this procedure, about 10 to 20 percent of the nucleus has been eliminated.

By reducing the nucleus, this procedure alleviates pressure on the disc and nerve roots. There is less risk to surrounding tissues because temperatures are considerably lower during this treatment method. The probe used in radiofrequency discal nucleoplasty can easily be compared to a microwave. It heats the object it is designed to heat but is not hot to the touch.

Still, it is important to consider the fact that this is a very new treatment option. In fact, radiofrequency discal nucleoplasty has been available for less than a year as of now. With new treatments such as this, it is crucial for both physicians and patients to keep up with current research on treatments in order to determine their effectiveness and whether any is right for you.

Consult Your Physician

If you suffer from back pain as a result of fissures located in one or more of your discs, IDET may be the best option for you. On the other hand, radiofrequency discal nucleoplasty is a cutting-edge technology treatment for decompressing a herniated disc. Moreover, its cooler temperature protects nearby tissues. The best way to know which option is best for you is to consult your physician. What's more, you should discuss non-invasive conservative therapies (pain medication, chiropractic care, etc.) before making the final decision to use one of these methods or any of the other invasive conservative remedies.

Decompression Surgery: The Differences Between Microdiscectomy and Open Discectomy and How They Affect Your Health

The decision to undergo surgery is usually a very difficult one. For most patients, it is their final attempt to find pain relief. There are still more options that can be explored to make the procedure less invasive. For instance, decompression surgery is among the most common procedures used to treat back pain. As surgery becomes more advanced, specialists are discovering more ways to make surgeries less invasive. This has certainly proven true when it comes to decompression surgery, also known as a discectomy (excision of a disc).

Discs are located in between the vertebrae along the spine. They are filled with a jelly-like fluid that is encased by a sturdy outer layer. However, an injury may cause the substance to overflow, pressing on nerves that are located nearby. This condition may result in sciatica, which occurs when a disc herniation presses on the sciatic nerve. This causes a shooting pain within the lower back and leg. For some patients, it makes standing unbearable. Others have difficulty raising the leg when they are lying flat. While 90 percent of patients recover from conservative treatment methods, some decide to explore spinal surgery.

More than likely, those patients who do not recover from conservative methods will undergo a discectomy, which is also known as decompression surgery. During a discectomy, the surgeon removes the disc herniation through a small incision, which is usually about two to five inches long.

Moreover, you may be eligible for a less invasive form of this surgical procedure. There are two main types of decompression surgery. If you are interested in receiving the least invasive form of discectomy, a microdiscectomy (microdecompression) may be an option for you.

In contrast to an open discectomy, a microdiscectomy has a smaller incision and does far less damage to nearby muscle tissue. For instance, during an open discectomy, also called a lumbar laminectomy, the surgeon will strip off the muscles that obstruct the path to the disc which needs to be excised.

However, during a microdiscectomy, these muscles are gently moved to the side. With these back muscles running vertically, it is not always necessary to cut them. Moreover, some surgeons use a tube-shaped retractor that tunnels through the muscles. This is also permissive for a smaller incision with no stripping away of the muscles. Needless to say, if you have no choice but to undergo spinal surgery, you will be better served by going with the least invasive procedure possible.

There are several advantages to choosing a microdiscectomy as opposed to an open discectomy. First of all, the recovery time is much faster. Patients who undergo a microdiscectomy may leave the hospital in as little as two hours or within 48 hours after the surgery. On the contrary, those who receive a lumbar laminectomy remain in the hospital for two to four days.

Yet, even if you opt for microdecompression surgery, there is still a chance you will have to undergo an open discectomy. For instance, the surgeon may decide that the muscles obstruct his view more than anticipated. If this is the case, he will resort to cutting and removing the muscle tissue after all. Nonetheless, there are some circumstances in which a surgeon will advocate a lumbar laminectomy in the first place.

For example, people with stenosis are typically candidates for this procedure. Patients who encounter stenosis usually experience pain brought on by a narrowing of the canal through which nerves pass along the spine. In most cases, this condition occurs in elderly people diagnosed with osteoarthritis, which is characterized by degeneration of the spine.

This degeneration results in larger facet joints and neighboring ligaments; this leaves less room for nerves to move freely along the spine, which leads to back pain. People with these conditions usually undergo a lumbar laminectomy due to the fact that bone is also extracted to relieve pressure over the nerve root. Therefore a larger incision is required during this operation.

Here is a brief description: The surgeon begins by making the incision and removing the lamina, which exposes the nerve roots. Then, the facet joints are trimmed. In some situations, a surgeon will also fuse the joints to keep the condition from recurring and also to stabilize the affected area. After the operation, it is highly recommended that patients walk; however, unnecessary bending, twisting, and lifting must be avoided for the first six weeks of recovery.

Fortunately, many patients find relief after their surgery. Some patients, however, will continue to experience some back pain as a result of other complications. For instance, if there is arthritis in the facet joints, this pain will remain unaffected by decompression surgery. For reasons such as these, surgery should always be a last resort.

If back pain can be managed through less invasive therapy, it certainly should be, especially since most of the conservative treatments will alleviate pain caused by multiple symptoms. For example, with chiropractic treatment, the practitioner will work on different areas of the spine simultaneously. Pain management techniques such as ultrasound and transcutaneous nerve stimulation can be used to treat several different areas.

Both microdiscectomy and lumbar laminectomy carry risks unique to surgical procedures. These include bleeding, infection, bladder incontinence, constipation, and dural tear. A dural tear results in the leaking of cerebrospinal fluid, which translates to a longer recovery time.

What You Should Know Before You Have Lumbar Fusion Surgery

Lumbar fusion surgery can be useful in treating serious illnesses that result in spinal deformity. It can help to stabilize a weak spine, allowing patients with debilitating conditions such as scoliosis and curvature of the spine to lead more active and fulfilling lifestyles. However, since there are so many risks with this procedure, it may not always be the best solution for treating back pain.

As with any spinal surgery, all conservative treatment options should be considered before lumbar fusion surgery. Still, if you are among the few patients with back pain who may benefit from this type of surgery, there is some information you must have beforehand. After all, when it comes to a procedure as serious as back surgery, you should be aware of your options and what you might expect.

When vertebrae move out of alignment and press on nerves within the spine, it can cause significant pain. In such cases, orthopedic surgeons rely on a procedure called lumbar fusion. This course of action is common in patients with spinal diseases such as spondylolisthesis (a displaced vertebra usually located in the lower back) and degenerative disc disease.

Some specialists recommend it as a means of alleviating back pain caused by sciatica, which pain from pressure on the sciatic nerve. Moreover, sciatica can cause severe back and leg pain. Nonetheless, spinal fusion surgery is used not only to treat back pain but also to correct deformities. For example, it is used to treat patients with deformities such as curvature of the spine, weakness in the spine caused by tumors, infection, or scoliosis.

In order to stabilize the vertebrae, a surgeon places bone grafts, screws, plates, or special cages where the damaged disc was prior to the surgery. Typically one of these materials is used to fashion bridges between the vertebrae. Using a bone graft to mend this area is preferred. If the situation is permissive, surgeons will take a bone graft from the patient's hip or pelvis.

Otherwise, they will obtain a bone graft from a bone bank. Using a bone graft from the patient's body allows the two vertebrae to become adjoined by a natural substance already present in the body. In most cases, there are fewer post-operative complications when a bone graft is taken from the patient. Additionally, synthetic bone grafts are currently in development for future use.

Once the treatment is complete, the vertebrae should be fused together and the area that was once causing so much pain should be left immobile, reducing the likelihood of back pain in the future. The result of this surgery should be that the vertebrae affixed to their proper positions. The irritated disc is completely eliminated from the patient's body and no longer able to inhibit that individual from enjoying a reasonably pain-free existence.

Still, lumbar fusion surgery works best when it is used for only one joint. Though it may be used for more than one, this greatly reduces mobility. There are few situations in which surgeons will perform more than one fusion and these typically do not involve pain management. Usually, they are situations that involve spinal weakness or deformity.

It is essential that patients who smoke stop doing so before they undergo lumbar fusion, as nicotine inhibits bone formation. It may be difficult to quit but there is no alternative if you would like to recover successfully. Meanwhile, some motion must be limited for the first three months after surgery, particularly bending, twisting, and lifting. Also, it is important to remember that there are several different types of lumbar fusion surgery.

Posterolateral Gutter Spine Fusion Surgery

This variation of lumbar fusion surgery is considered the "tried and true" method. During this procedure, the surgeon begins by extracting a bone graft from the pelvis, working with the same incision she will use to perform the fusion. This incision is located on the patient's back.

Next, the bone graft is placed on the outside of the spine in a very vascular area. This environment is especially conducive to bone production due to the healthful circulation of nutrient-rich blood. Lastly, muscles that were raised up in order to provide a bed for the bone graft are lowered onto it. The tension in these muscles helps to keep the graft in place.

Posterior Lumbar Interbody Fusion (PLIF)

Like posterolateral gutter spine surgery, the incision is made in the patient's back. Then, the laminae are stripped in order to reveal the nerve roots. If necessary, the facet joints are trimmed in order to ease pressure on the nerve roots. Once the nerve roots have been moved aside, the disc is cleaned so that the bone graft can be inserted directly into the disc space.

Anterior Lumbar Interbody Fusion (ALIF)

This procedure is very similar to PLIF except that it is achieved through the abdomen rather than the back. Thus, this method has a couple of advantages such as greater ease in removing the disc space in addition to the ability to insert a much larger bone graft, However, this procedure is insufficient when dealing with a great deal of instability. If the spine is unstable, it may be best to combine posterior and anterior lumbar fusion surgery.

Transforaminal Lumbar Interbody Fusion (TLIF)

TLIF is basically a newer and more improved version of PLIF. For instance, during PLIF, a portion of each facet joint is removed. In contrast, during a TLIF, one entire facet joint is removed, which increases visibility and allows the surgeon to remove a larger amount of disc material. However, the ALIF is still the best method for optimal visualization, access to disc space, and more surface area for healing. Still, the ALIF is usually used along with the PLIF, which means that the patient must recover from two incisions rather than just one.

Of course, as with any surgery, there are drawbacks. The most important point to consider as a patient is that the drawbacks with lumbar fusion surgery are fairly severe. First and foremost, only about 60 percent of those who endure this operation can expect to be alleviated of their back pain. Also, though all surgeries come with certain risks, there are several potentially serious side effects that could occur after spinal fusion surgery.

For example, there is a risk of increased stress on remaining discs, in particular those adjacent to the fused vertebrae. Unfortunately, this could lead to complications in the future. Moreover, some patients develop a distended abdomen, which prevents them from eating; a special tube may be necessary in order to correct it.

In addition to this post-operative correction, people who experience lumbar fusion surgery may have to go through additional procedures. In some cases, they encounter pain at the fusion site, most often when they have received a bone graft from a donor. If the fusion is unable to heal properly, more surgery may be required. Also, fusions held together by screws, rods, plates, or any other hardware are subject to its breakability. This type of complication may also lead to additional surgery. Nevertheless, as with any surgical procedure, there is also a possibility of bleeding and infection as well as urinary tract infections and urinary retention.

The Newest Developments in Spinal Surgery and Whether You Should Consider Them

There are many different invasive and non-invasive back pain treatments that members of the medical community would consider to be tried and true. Many of these treatment methods have been improved upon with the advancement of technology. For example, instead of an open discectomy, many surgeons will perform a microdiscectomy, which is less invasive.

Most importantly, as physicians continue to learn about back pain and conservative treatment options, these non-invasive methods become more effective. This is great news for patients because it means that more people rely on conservative treatments and are not forced to undergo spinal surgery. For those who are in need of surgery, there are different options available and all are worth checking into beforehand.

As surgeons move toward less invasive procedures, breakthrough procedures are emerging. Not only are they emerging, they are being used throughout the world. Two of the latest spinal surgery procedures include Kyphoplasty, which is usually used to correct spinal deformity, and lumbar artificial disc surgery, an alternative to lumbar fusion surgery.

Kyphoplasty

This type of surgery is common among patients diagnosed with compression fractures as well as those suffering from osteoporosis, the loss of calcium in the bones that causes small holes throughout the vertebrae. Furthermore, this procedure is more common among patients with osteoporosis who do not find pain relief from medication, bracing, or other passive conservative therapies.

Most people think of osteoporosis as a condition characterized by fractures of the bone. However, the vertebrae of a person with osteoporosis have pore-like holes. This disease does more than just cause shrinkage or a "hump" that may appear depending on the severity of an individual case. It also causes chronic back pain, decreased mobility, diminished lung capacity, and difficulty sleeping. Thus, people with osteoporosis encounter an overall loss of independence and loss of ability to perform daily pursuits.

The purpose of kyphoplasty is to prevent deformities and back pain caused by the breakage. Here is how it works: First, the surgeon makes two small incisions in the patient's skin. Then, he or she places a balloon in each of the incisions. Once placed, each balloon is inflated, expanding the bone back to a normal size. And finally, the newly opened space is filled with liquid cement.

Many osteopathic surgeons prefer kyphoplasty over its precursor, which is called vertebroplasty. This earlier surgical practice is the same as kyphoplasty but without the balloon to keep the liquid cement from leaking into the bloodstream. Though an incident such as this is very rare, it must be taken seriously.

If the cement were to contaminate the bloodstream, it would create new pressure on the spinal cord; thus, emergency decompression surgery would be necessary. Moreover, there is some risk due to the fact that the repaired vertebra becomes hardened as the liquid cement sets in. As a result, neighboring vertebrae are put under increased pressure. Unfortunately, this could even create fractures in the nearby vertebrae.

Lumbar Artificial Disc Surgery

This procedure has become very popular in Europe and is turning into a preferred surgical method for alleviating chronic back pain in the U.S. Though lumbar fusion is usually the surgeon's choice for treating chronic back pain, more surgeons in the U.S. are beginning to explore lumbar artificial disc surgery to provide pain relief.

One key advantage of this procedure over lumbar fusion is that lumbar artificial disc surgery allows the patient to maintain natural spine movement. Proponents of this surgery believe that sustaining normal motion will decrease the likelihood of Transition Syndrome, which is characterized by the premature degeneration at adjacent levels of the spine.

When a patient undergoes a spinal fusion procedure, the joints that are adjacent to the fused joints may be forced to take on additional stress. This is due to the decreased mobility occurring at the fused area. Furthermore, there are two main varieties of lumbar artificial disc surgery; thus, one replaces only the nucleus of a disc while the other replaces the entire disc. Of course, disc nucleus replacement surgery is still in the investigation phase here in the U.S. Meanwhile, it is being performed in other countries worldwide.

Is Surgery Really Best?

Many people who receive back surgery often expect to wake up cured or feel total relief after the recommended recovery period. However, it is important to remember that back pain most often can not be cured. Instead, it can only be managed.

Before considering spinal surgery, you should always try non-invasive or minimally invasive conservative methods before going under the knife. After all, there is a very good chance that passive treatment such as massage therapy or chiropractic adjustments will help manage the pain in the same way (or even better) than back surgery.

Furthermore, chiropractic treatment and physical therapy help treat the root cause of back pain rather than simply covering it up, which is the only way to truly ensure permanent or at least long-term relief from back pain. It is essential that all patients regard surgery as an absolute last resort.

Alternative Treatments

The Mechanism of Acupuncture

Acupuncture is an age-old technique first used in China thousands of years ago. It involves the use of specialized, stainless steel needles, which are inserted in various locations of the body. These locations are called "acupuncture points" and specific combinations are used to stimulate healing. Commonly known as an alternative treatment approach, acupuncture is becoming increasingly popular in North America.

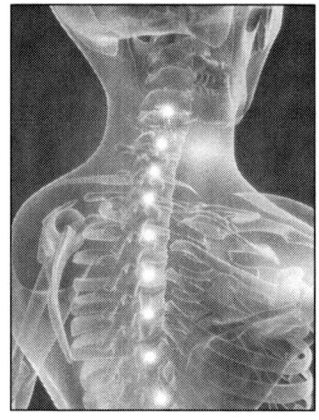

Although acupuncture is relatively new to Western culture, it is becoming a very viable treatment option for pain. The technique has been the subject of several studies which seem to indicate that acupuncture does provide significant relief for individuals who present with chronic pain syndromes, especially those with back pain. For detailed information see http://www.umm.edu/news/releases/back_pain.htm where subjects with varying degrees of lower back pain experienced relief after treatment with acupuncture.

What Is The Theory Behind Acupuncture for Back Pain?

The foundations of traditional Chinese medicine are based on the belief that everyone possesses an individual and specific energy flow, or qi. If the qi becomes unbalanced or blocked, illness or disease is the result.

Yin and yang are part of qi, and represent the whole energy force that work together to maintain the necessary balance of energy required for the body to function. If there is too much of one or not enough of the other, the body's energy flow, or qi, is disrupted and can cause any number of symptoms or conditions, with back pain one of them.

Acupuncture utilizes a combination of thin, specialized needles to help direct qi through a series of channels in the body called meridians. These are found in pairs representing each side of the body and are essentially the pathways by which the energy flows throughout the body.

The needles are placed in position along specific meridians in order to help the qi move freely throughout the body thus removing any blockages or gaps in the energy flow. Thus back pain according to the ancient Chinese medicine theory is caused by these interruptions in qi and once it is restored and able to move freely anywhere in the body, the pain is alleviated.

Endorphins and Acupuncture: Working Together

Before trying acupuncture to help relieve back pain, it is helpful to learn exactly how the body responds and what to expect from it. Most research suggests that there is a process initiated when acupuncture needles are inserted in the body.

The body, and more specifically the brain, interprets the positioning of the acupuncture needles as a stimulus to the peripheral nervous system. It responds by immediately releasing endorphins to the nerve pathways.

Endorphins are the body's own pain-killing compounds that work to block the pain pathways from the brain to the affected areas. The result is an all natural treatment for pain. Acupuncture seems to provide a relatively quick and effective way to reduce or eliminate pain where the body itself is called to action as it sends relief to the areas of the body in need of help.

When endorphins are able to provide symptom relief, there may be more options available for a patient in pain. In some cases, acupuncture may work in combination with other treatment methods to help those suffering with back pain.

The Treatment Plan: What to Expect

Typical treatment for back pain with acupuncture may be determined by many factors. Relief may be immediate or may require a series of treatment sessions to control or eliminate the symptoms. Once the patient is evaluated by a professionally trained acupuncturist, the treatment plan may be determined.

During the initial visit, the acupuncturist will require complete medical history including any previous conditions as well as your current health status. Specific symptoms will be discussed as well as the severity and length of each. Patient progress is monitored as they will be asked to report response and any improvement during and after each session.

The acupuncturist will explain how the technique works and what it will feel like when the needles are used. Usually, a treatment session lasts about an hour and is required once or twice a week. The length of treatment varies but, generally, the course of treatment consists of 10 to 12 acupuncture sessions.

The Future of Acupuncture in Western Medicine

Acupuncture is becoming a much more accepted and proven method for treating a number of conditions. From back pain to sports injuries and cancer, acupuncture can often be a very useful and effective treatment option. Still considered alternative, this technique continues to gain momentum as more and more people experience the benefits of acupuncture.

Despite the fact that the benefits of acupuncture are gaining worldwide attention, complimentary medicine is still considered "new" in North America where Western traditional medicine has always been the norm. But as some current studies suggest, acupuncture is proving to be an effective treatment for many conditions and especially pain relief.

For the patient who has sought many kinds of treatment for back pain without success, acupuncture may be just what the doctor ordered.

Herbal Medicine and Back Pain

The Evolution of Herbal Medicine

Medicinal herbs have been used for thousands of years by ancient peoples worldwide. Everyone is familiar with reports of the village "medicine man" or "shaman" who would administer special combinations of herbs and other natural remedies to treat any kind of condition. There are over 6000 herbs in existence and many have been found to be very effective in treating a wide range of afflictions.

Herbs, as a whole, are derived from plant products and have many uses. Some are used to enhance the flavor of food while others are found to be very effective for medicinal purposes.

Illness and disease have been present since the beginning of time and so has the need for identification and treatment to ensure survival and to maintain existence. While searching for food and other necessities, primitive cultures tried many kinds of plants found in their surroundings. They noticed that some made them ill but others had unique effects that actually improved existing conditions and made them stronger and healthier. From generation to generation, these herbs were used to treat ailments and as more and more were discovered, the ability of the local "healers" became more specific and useful.

Recently, there has been increased interest in the effects of herbal medicine for a variety of ailments. With such a wide range of herbal remedies available, there seems to be something for virtually every condition known to Western medicine. Both chronic and acute back pain may be treated with various forms of herbal medicine with positive results.

Using Medicinal Herbs Safely

Before starting any herbal medicine, remember to consult an accredited healthcare provider. She can explain the purpose of the herbs recommended as well as the benefits for your back pain. Be certain that you are clear and don't hesitate to ask any questions or address any concerns you may have about the treatment plan.

Make a list of all medications you are currently taking including pharmaceuticals prescribed by your doctor as well as any herbal remedies. Check with your healthcare provider to determine if there could be any drug interactions as you add new herbs to your treatment protocol.

Take the herbal medications exactly as instructed and do not adjust the doses on your own. Report any changes in your condition, positive or negative, regularly. Your herbalist needs to monitor your response and make any changes or adjustments as necessary.

Herbal medicine can be a safe and effective treatment for back pain. Studies show that certain herbs are very helpful in alleviating pain. When used in specific combinations and under the care of a qualified professional, herbal medicine may be just what you need for your back pain.

Which Herbs Are Used to Treat Back Pain?

Often, combinations of medicinal herbs are used to treat back pain symptoms. Some of the most specific for pain, inflammation and joints are willow bark, devil's claw, valerian, and cayenne.

Willow Bark   Originating from a tree found in Europe, the leaves of the willow bark contain a substance called "salicin" which has been found to reduce pain and inflammation.

Devil's Claw   Found in Africa, Devil's Claw is named for the tiny "hooks" on the fruit of the plant. The active ingredient in Devil's Claw is "iridoid glycosides" which is often effective for inflammation and pain including back, neck, and arthritic symptoms.

Valerian Root   This plant exists in North and South America, Europe and Asia and is most commonly used to treat insomnia but is also credited for its anti-spasmodic properties as well as a muscle relaxant.

Cayenne   An ingredient in cayenne peppers, "capsaicin" is often used in a cream which is applied to the affected area. It seems to "dull" pain as the body responds by reducing the pain sensation. As the effect is only temporary, the cream must be re-applied at intervals.

The Benefits of Herbs for Back Pain

Because herbal remedies are usually considered less toxic than most pharmaceutical drugs, and consist of all-natural ingredients, they are generally better tolerated with fewer side effects. For those who suffer from back pain, this may be a low risk but beneficial treatment option.

Medicinal herbs work differently than synthetic drugs since pharmaceuticals treat individual symptoms while herbs focus on the underlying conditions causing the symptoms. Since herbal remedies are less toxic, they can be used over longer periods of time than synthetic drugs. For long-term or chronic back pain, herbs may be used safely until relief is achieved.

Herbs help with pain and inflammation by restoring the body's natural state of wellness. Herbal treatment acts as a stimulus for the individual's own body to initiate healing and promote whole-body wellness and balance. As a result, the remedies work to relieve your back pain and other imbalances that may be contributing to your condition.

Herbal medicine has been used by many cultures since the beginning of time. As the knowledge base and case-study information continues to grow, so does the recognition of this form of treatment for many conditions, including back pain and its related symptoms. Studies show positive results with herbal treatment for all kinds of pain and it does seem to be a worthy option for those suffering from the effects of back pain.

What Is The Attraction? Magnetic Therapy for Back Pain

When dealing with back pain, any form of relief is appreciated. Magnetic therapy is becoming one of the most recommended alternative treatment methods and is gaining plenty of positive attention for its effectiveness in pain relief. The ideology behind this increasingly popular approach is relatively easy to understand and has many applications.

Magnetic therapy is non-invasive and is relatively cost effective compared to other forms of treatment available for back pain sufferers. Plus, many patients notice improvement in their pain after only a few sessions.

The use of magnets for healing is not new. The practice has been in use for thousands of years but is now gaining recognition in a variety of settings for its profound effect on pain and inflammation.

What Is Magnetic Therapy?

Magnetic therapy involves placing special high powered magnets on the body where there is pain, inflammation, muscle tension, or tissue damage. The magnets act as stimuli which activate the body's own healing response. The magnets may be placed in various locations or directly on the affected area.

The Principles: Healing with Magnets

According to the basic theory of magnetic healing, the body possesses a unique form of energy. This energy is what scientists call "bioelectricity" and consists of the electrical charge found in every cell of the body.

When the body's energy is unbalanced, blocked or damaged, magnets can be applied to the affected areas. The magnets help to correct the energy and stimulate healing.

Magnets operate using positive and negative pulls where opposites attract. Since blood contains a small percentage of iron, which is attracted by magnetic pull, magnets placed on the body cause a unique and positive effect. When the negative side of a magnet is applied to any affected area of the body, it attracts positive and healthy new blood. This creates a balanced magnetic response which increases circulation, and reduces inflammation and pain.

Patients often experience an immediate reduction in pain levels as well as an increased sense of energy. Magnetic therapy is also reported to improve the amount of quality sleep where patients previously suffered from interrupted and restless sleep patterns.

What to Expect from Magnetic Therapy for Your Back Pain

Whether you choose to receive magnetic therapy in an alternative healthcare provider's office or use specialized magnetic pads that you wear on your body, you can benefit from the amazing effect of magnets.

Many people report almost instant relief of their back pain after wearing magnetized back pads while others use magnetic mattresses for relief at night and more restful sleep. While each case differs, relief from back pain is possible within a reasonably short treatment period.

Magnetic therapy is safe, non-invasive and non toxic. There are no side effects and it is much more cost-effective than many other treatment options for back pain. And since magnetic therapy creates a more balanced flow of energy throughout the entire body, patients may experience overall wellness and improvement in other symptoms as well.

Patients who have experienced magnetic therapy often report:

- ❖ Significant pain relief
- ❖ Improved circulation
- ❖ Reduced inflammation
- ❖ Healing and tissue repair
- ❖ Reduced muscle pain/stiffness
- ❖ More restful sleep

With such noted improvement and recovery from so many common back-related symptoms, magnetic therapy has plenty to offer sufferers.

Try Magnetic Therapy for Your Own Back Pain

Although treatment for back pain may be given in an alternative healthcare setting, many products are available in a variety of forms for those interested in utilizing magnetic therapy at home.

Mattresses/Pads Specially designed mattresses and/or pads consist of magnets placed in various parts so that you can get the benefits of magnetic therapy while you sleep.

Magnetic Wraps and Supports   Used to relieve pain, magnetic wraps are placed around the affected area and consist of magnets woven into the fabric. When placed on the back, the magnets help to lessen or eliminate symptoms.

Spot Magnets   Placed on the back for specific time periods, the effects of the magnets can give much needed improvement in back pain. Since the spot magnets can be placed in various locations on the back, they can directly target problem areas for faster relief.

Back Braces   For severe or widespread back pain, a magnetic back brace may be a good idea. As well as providing the healing of magnets in the brace itself, it may also help to reduce more damage by keeping your back well supported.

Magnets: Positive Treatment for a Negative Condition

Back pain is one of the top reasons for visits to healthcare providers and continues to be one of the most common conditions affecting millions of people every day. Whether it is acute or chronic back pain, magnetic therapy has been shown to be a very promising treatment.

As magnetic therapy continues to gain acceptance, more and more people may be willing to experience the incredible benefits of magnets and how they can be used to treat back pain and related symptoms.

Bodywork for Back Pain

What Is Bodywork?

Bodywork is an approach to healing that emphasizes balance of body, mind and spirit through physical manipulation and movement. There are many variations of technique with specific method and treatment style. Generally, they all focus on whole body relaxation and harmony.

The ultimate goal is to increase awareness of how closely the mind and body work together for optimum wellness. When the mind is stressed and tense, so is the body. This would explain why we may experience a range of physical symptoms, such as back pain, during times of increased stress and mental strain.

Techniques Used Most Often in Bodywork Therapy

Some of the most common types of bodywork are massage, deep tissue manipulation, movement awareness, energy balancing, and trigger point therapy. Each one offers a unique form of therapy where the patient learns how to achieve less discomfort, more ease of movement, and an overall increase in energy.

Massage One of the most popular bodywork techniques for back pain is massage. It promotes both healing and muscle relaxation through physical manipulation. The massage therapist uses lotions or oils to aid in the ease of movement as they apply pressure to various muscles. As the tense, sore muscles are essentially "smoothed out" by the massage therapist, endorphins are released from the brain that help the patient relax and release tension in both body and mind as well as reduce pain.

Deep Tissue Manipulation This method of bodywork involves manipulation of problems areas with focus on the tissue surrounding muscles that can become stiff or inflamed. The therapist looks for areas where the muscles are tight, tense, or painful, and he kneads the area in order to reach the deep tissues. The result is better blood flow to the area, pain relief, and improved muscle movement.

Movement Awareness Unlike massage or deep tissue manipulation, movement awareness focuses on teaching the patient to become more aware of his or her own body movement. Various kinds of exercises are used in which the patient is asked to move as they would normally everyday. This may be how they bend to pick up an object or walk across a room. The therapist will work with the patient to determine which movement may be aggravating the muscles of the back and how to make changes to eliminate it.

Energy Balancing Based on the belief that the entire universe operates under many kinds and forms of energy, the methods used in energy balancing centre on one's own ability and desire to use this energy to balance all function in the body. An energy healer helps to stimulate the process with a "hands-on" approach.

The patient lies down and the therapist gently massages the areas where excessive stress and tension are causing the energy imbalance. There may be a sense of warmth or coolness, relaxation, or overall calmness as well. The individual's own energy interacts with the universal energy to create a balance that relieves the pain and tension.

Trigger Point Therapy Also referred to as myotherapy, trigger point therapy is often useful for back pain. The therapist works with the patient to determine specific areas where the pain, inflammation, and tense muscles are present. They apply pressure on these areas directly to relieve the symptoms.

Once the patient's trigger points are found, the therapist teaches the patient how to move and stretch the muscles so that ongoing relief is maintained. In the event of a relapse, the patient is also encouraged to find someone at home to learn the locations of the trigger points so that immediate therapy may be given if symptoms start to recur.

Bodywork and Back Pain

With such a varied number of bodywork techniques available for your back pain, you may decide to try a few of them to determine which ones are the most effective for you. All of the methods offer a wide range of benefits and symptom relief for both short- and long-term back ailments.

Your back pain may be more than just an isolated symptom. As the rationale behind bodywork suggests, the back pain may be connected to mental stress or overwork. The key to correcting symptoms that arise is to acknowledge this and achieve overall wellness where you learn to recognize how your mind, body, and spirit must all be in balance. Your mental state may be adding to your physical symptoms as your body reacts by causing back pain or other symptoms.

Since bodywork techniques address both physical and mental awareness and how they relate to whole body wellness, the patient's improvement may be seen as all-encompassing healing where balance between body and mind is restored. The relief of pain, muscle stiffness, and tightness is paired with increased energy, relaxation, and mental alertness. This leads to an overall boost to the immune system as the tension and stress are alleviated. When all of these things occur in harmony, wellness and freedom from back pain (and its triggers) are the result.

Pilates: The Gentle Way to Deal with Back Pain

Introduced in the early 1900s by Joseph Pilates, the Pilates exercise fitness program was invented while Pilates was in a German interment camp during World War I. He taught his fellow interns the various exercises to help them maintain their wellness and to make their bodies more resistant to illness. After the war, he immigrated to New York City where he and his wife opened a studio to teach the Pilates method.

The Pilates method is becoming increasingly popular and is gaining worldwide attention for its unique approach to whole body fitness and wellness without building muscle bulk. Unlike other exercise regimens, Pilates is a much gentler, soothing form of body conditioning that may be useful for many conditions, including back pain and injury.

Pilates Exercises Are Very Spine-related

Major emphasis in Pilates training is its benefit to the spine. The exercises offered are gentle and help to strengthen muscles of the back and spine. Pilates believed that the abdominal area was the centre of the body's function and strength there would have a ripple effect to the rest of the body. Exercises that improved posture and breathing would reduce stress on the spine. This would create stronger torso muscles and thus lead to more support for the back. All of this would work together to lead the body to a complete, well balanced state of wellness.

The spine is the central structure that is designed to support the rest of the body. Due to overwork, prolonged periods of sitting or simple lack of exercise, the spine may become too curved or out of alignment. This leads to back pain, stiffness, and poor posture.

Pilates exercises address these problems with focus on strengthening and stretching the muscles that surround the spine, back, and neck. Breathing routines teach more effective ways to ensure that our abdominal and chest muscles are working so that there is less pressure on the back and spine.

Stretch, Strengthen, and Balance

Core components of the Pilates program are ways to make all parts of the body work with each other smoothly and effectively for optimum performance and wellness. This is done through the specially designed exercises developed by Pilates. Muscles are stretched and strengthened without heavy, intense exercise, while at the same time balancing the body and mind.

The abdominal area is the central focus of the Pilates method. It is called "the powerhouse" because Pilates thought that muscles found in this area and the spine are the most important. Developing exercises that would strengthen and stretch these muscles would provide a central support from which the rest of the body could benefit.

Who Should Try Pilates?

Just about anyone, young or old, physically conditioned or new to any fitness program, can improve by trying the Pilates method. Because it involves mild but powerful exercise routines, people in almost any physical condition can be successful. There is no jumping, lifting, or bouncing involved that may be too harsh or demanding for some people.

Dancers are particularly attracted to Pilates since the method emphasizes stretching, balance, and improved breathing exercises for muscles without adding bulk. Pilates promotes flexibility and ease of movement which are also essential in dance.

Both the elderly and overweight can also find that Pilates is useful since it does not require intense physical activity such as aerobics or cardiovascular routines. Pilates offers slow, calming, and relaxing movement that is not stressful or highly exertive.

Healing with Pilates

Pilates is one of the few exercise techniques that can be used for rehabilitation and to accelerate healing. A fitness program for those recovering from injury requires safe yet productive exercise, and Pilates has both.

Recovery from soft tissue injury is often possible when an appropriate Pilates regimen is implemented and adapted as the individual improves and regains movement and function. This is especially the case for many suffering from back pain and injury. Starting slowly and with a conservative exercise plan, Pilates can make back muscles more flexible and stronger. There is also benefit to the spine as the muscles begin to provide more support.

In addition to the healing ability in Pilates, the method remains flexible enough that it can be personalized to any kind of injury or condition. A Pilates trainer can work with the client to determine which combination of exercises would be most effective for their particular situation. For example, some people who require rehabilitation from surgery or a prolonged illness can find the Pilates program that works well for them.

Perhaps the reason Pilates has become so widely used in a variety of settings today is because of its unique ability to adapt to the needs of its users. There is no set textbook protocol that must be followed by everyone taking part in the program. The exercises promote relaxation and balance for both body and mind. And there is no demanding, high-stress activity, so that people can work at their own pace and ability while still achieving healing and wellness.

Rolfing: Unlock The Body from Back Pain

It may be time to try Rolfing to rid your body of the aches and pain that affect your back and muscles. Developed by Dr. Ida Rolf in the 1950s, Rolfing is also known as "Structural Integration" and is becoming a popular exercise program.

Basic Theory Behind The Rolfing Method

The technique is very straightforward and is based on the assumption that the body is designed to be structured and aligned with the centre of gravity. Due to a lifestyle that doesn't include regular exercise but does involve long periods of sitting (at work, on the sofa…), the body begins to become unbalanced with poor posture. This also adds stress to the muscles and other connective tissue, which results in an assortment of ailments, including back pain.

According to Rolfing theory, the connective tissue that covers muscles, called "fascia", becomes lumped together and misshapen. When this happens, the muscles can no longer function the way in which they were intended. The result is stress, pain, and loss of posture.

The purpose of the Rolfing method is to break down or "unlock" the "fascia" or connective tissue, smooth out, and rebuild muscles. Once the muscles are able to work freely again, posture is improved and users regain much more ease in movement. The body is re-structured and the muscles can work much more efficiently in alignment with gravity.

Rolfing: The Ten Series

The Rolfing program consists of 10 one-hour sessions called the "ten series" where each is designed to focus on specific muscles and areas of the body. After the initial program, there are "tune up" programs where Rolfers can revisit familiar exercises and maintain their own workout regime.

Each exercise involves soft tissue manipulation with special attention to connective tissue. The goal is to provide appropriate exercises for the entire body where the premise is that pain or discomfort in one area may be caused by problems in another part of the body. For example, shoulder and back pain may be caused by poor posture and alignment problems in the legs.

The sessions are designed to build on each other where there is focus on different layers of connective tissue in each one. The first three sessions involve work with the superficial layers. Better breathing is encouraged through exercises for the muscles around the lungs, ribcage, and pelvis. The next three sessions move to deeper layers and include exercises for the legs, abdomen, back, and hips. The remaining sessions offer techniques for integrating all of the previous sessions and using them for overall body function.

Rolfing Back Pain Away

While you may be willing to try Rolfing for your back pain, there may be much more to gain than you first thought. Since the Rolfing theory associates whole body wellness with each one of its principles, the program may correct your back pain and other ailments too. The back pain may be a prominent symptom but may be occurring in conjunction with problems in other areas of your body.

Rolfing exercises can correct and repair the fascia in muscles of your back, abdomen, legs, neck, and pelvis which all work together to support your spine.

As the spine is regarded as the structure that is the centre of balance and from which gravity is aligned, the Rolfing program provides the exercises needed to relieve your back pain and contribute to a greater quality of wellness. The effects of gravity on the body can be seen in poor posture and abnormal curve in the spine from prolonged imbalance. This causes increased gravitational pull that puts improper and unnecessary stress on muscles, tendons, ligaments, joints, and fascia. The body responds by exhibiting painful symptoms including tense, stiff, inflamed and rigid soft tissue.

Benefits for Both Body and Mind

As well as the physical exercises to improve overall body wellness, the Rolfing method also incorporates psychological benefits too. Rolfing teaches that hardened, tense fascia retains the effects of past injuries or emotional trauma. These can also cause a whole body stiffness or rigidity.

They are called "hot spots" and are just as important as the areas where the pain and discomfort are current. As the sessions are completed, Rolfing exercises address all of these areas so that a complete, balanced sense of well being is achieved and maintained.

Incorporating Rolfing into your plan to gain relief from back pain may yield many more positive results than you thought possible or even expected. Many users of the program report:

- ❖ Ease of movement
- ❖ Pain relief
- ❖ Increased flexibility
- ❖ Better posture
- ❖ Less muscle tension and stiffness
- ❖ Release of emotional issues
- ❖ Reduced stress

With so many advantages of Rolfing, there may be plenty to offer anyone who suffers from back pain. Learning how body structure and balance affect every system can be very useful as you begin to see the improvement in both body and mind with the Rolfing program.

Yoga: Uniting the Body, Mind and Spirit

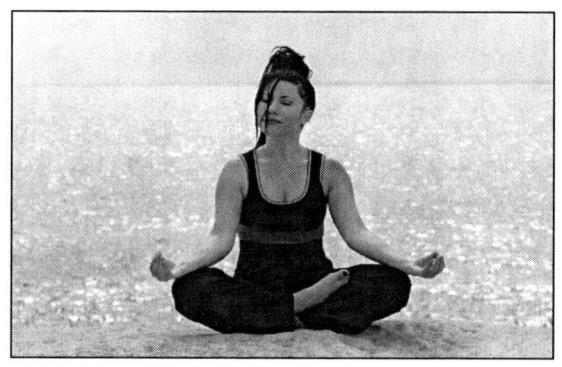

Have you ever considered yoga for back pain? It can help strengthen and stretch the spine so that the back muscles are no longer stressed and weakened. The benefits to your overall well being are an added incentive to create a more positive, balanced outlook that can enhance your entire being.

The roots of yoga begin literally thousands of years ago in ancient civilizations and exist today with great influence from Hindu teachings. The word, "yoga" is from ancient Sanskrit and means "unite" or "union" where basic principles of yoga are uniting the body, mind and spirit.

Although there have been several variations of yoga throughout the centuries, the basic teachings have essentially remained the same. The goal is to lead a well balanced, pleasant, and fulfilling life where students of yoga strive to attain ultimate freedom. There is no ego in yoga, so no one is considered better than anyone else. Each person must follow his own quest as he moves through the experience of living.

Practice Can Help with Back Pain

When most people think of yoga, they assume it is a fitness method requiring its students to perform all kinds of stretching and bending exercises that would be rather difficult for most people to master. In fact, there may be some truth in that assumption but yoga is much more than that.

Yoga teaches whole body, mind, and spirit health where each individual's journey is unique. A student of yoga develops at her own pace where the personal progress is called "your practice" and describes that student's experience over time.

Relief from back pain begins with the mental, physical, and spiritual principles of yoga. The physical aspect is described as a series of "poses" that provide specific benefits. They may be practiced quickly as a workout of sorts or slowly to incorporate the calming, relaxing attributes of traditional yoga. Most people looking for relief from back pain may opt for a combination of the physical and mental exercises to control the pain. This would include slow, gentle movement and meditation to stimulate the mind and strengthen the back at the same time.

Physical Rewards for Your Back

There are many benefits of yoga for your back pain. The kinds of exercises and "poses" stimulate healing and can help with both long-term pain issues and acute injuries. As you continue your practice, the effects may become long-lasting and can improve your whole body wellness.

Improved Breathing Techniques   One of the first kinds of exercises learned in yoga is how to breathe more effectively. Proper breathing requires that the body be upright and in position to allow as much fresh, oxygenated air into the body as possible. Regular breathing exercises also help with the lungs and abdominal muscles which in turn relieve pressure on the spine and pain in the back area.

Strengthens and Makes Muscles More Flexible   When practicing yoga, the key benefit for muscle strength and flexibility is to achieve and hold the pose. More experienced yogis can hold and sustain the exercise for longer periods of time while others who are using yoga to aid in recovery from injury or pain may need to practice with short holding exercises. Muscles in the back and abdomen are very important for support of the spine. When these muscles build strength, pressure is eased on the spine and pain is lessened or eliminated.

Stretching Improves Circulation and Muscle Function   Yoga poses and postures require significant forms of stretching exercises where the holding increases the blood flow to and from the muscles. Fresh, oxygenated blood flows to the muscles and more toxic, unhealthy blood moves out of the area. As circulation becomes more efficient, the muscles benefit through improved muscle function. Improved muscles in the legs, pelvis, and abdomen can help pain in the lower back.

Maintains the Natural Curvature of the Spine   Due to poor posture which occurs over a period of time when there is little exercise, extra weight, and frequent sitting, the spine may become stressed and misaligned. When this happens, the spine can no longer support or function as it was intended and the body responds with pain, changes in walking, and fatigue. Yoga exercises encourage stretching and balancing the body which also improves posture and helps the spine return to its proper curvature.

Mental Benefits of Yoga

Meditation   A well balanced, relaxed mental state is one of the cornerstones of yoga teaching. Physical exercise is important but so is the mental aspect. Once the student is able to attain a calm, soothing state of mind, they are able to meditate. Meditation allows the student to release stress, let go of any anxiety, or issue bothering them, and simply focus on positive, healing thoughts.

Mind Over Matter   Simply put, the mental and emotional release achieved through yoga exercise and meditation can contribute to a pain-free, healthy body. Many yogis believe that negative thinking can actually create or worsen physical symptoms. So believing that your back pain will continue to worsen and become disabling may be a self-fulfilling prophecy. Through positive thinking and meditation, you may be able to change how your body responds to minor back ailments, stress, and emotional triggers of back pain.

Chiropractic Care Can Stop Pain and Help Restore Good Health

The Philosophy of Chiropractic

To grasp the philosophy of chiropractic, you must first understand that chiropractic does not *have* a philosophy. Rather, chiropractic *is* a philosophy, as well as a science and an art. Chiropractic is not simply a treatment to adjust one's spine. It is, fundamentally, a set of beliefs about the human body and the natural order of our universe.

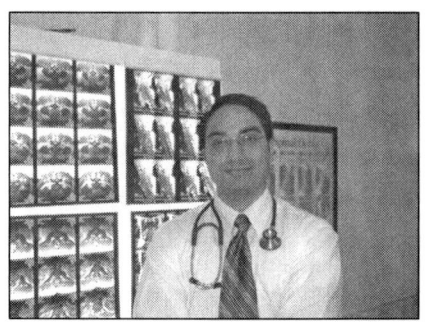

The foundation of chiropractic is built upon the vitalistic principle, which is a belief that the human body has the ability to keep itself healthy if there are no barriers to the full expression of all the body's vital functions. Put simply, chiropractic embraces the belief that the body has an innate ability to heal itself from within.

This innate knowledge is the vital force that not only allows the body to heal itself, but also helps us adapt naturally to both internal and external environmental influences.

For example, as the temperature outside rises, the body responds with perspiration to cool itself down. If the temperature is cold outside, the body takes measures to maintain its internal warmth. Every significant change in our external environment triggers a corresponding reaction in our bodies.

But what about the body's internal environment? Think of what happens when you get a virus. Your body interprets that virus as an invader and responds by raising your internal temperature (running a fever) and increasing waste elimination. This is your body's way of adapting to a significant change in its internal environment in order to restore its natural, healthy functions.

Symptoms Are Not The Enemy

Chiropractic understands that a symptom is not a disease, nor should it be treated as one.

In actuality, a symptom functions as an "alarm bell" of sorts, advising you of a barrier or obstacle in your body's ability to heal and maintain itself. Many times, this alarm (the symptom) is the only way for you to know that something is amiss with your body.

At the heart of the chiropractic philosophy is a steadfast belief in treating the root cause of the problem, not just the symptoms. When you address only the symptoms, the underlying problem remains and will continue manifesting itself until it is corrected.

Instead, chiropractic recognizes symptoms as normal adaptive bodily functions and avoids the use of medications or treatments that force the body to react in a way contrary to its built-in ability to heal itself. In most cases, medication merely masks the symptoms while doing nothing at all to heal the actual underlying problem.

Oftentimes, the real problem can arise in the *absence* of symptoms. How often have you been shocked to learn that someone has passed away quite suddenly and unexpectedly? Your first thought might be, "But he was so healthy and didn't seem to ever get sick." Obviously, this person did not enjoy such glowing good health, and he was probably sick considerably more often than was apparent.

Without symptoms, we remain ignorant of the barriers and interferences that can impede our health, sometimes until the damage becomes too severe. Our bodies do not have infinite abilities to adapt and heal. But even though we cannot expand the finite limitations of our bodies, there is a great deal we can do through chiropractic care to eliminate artificial barriers to our good health.

So listen to your body, particularly when symptoms manifest. And even if you feel perfectly healthy, it is a wise person who actively maintains the innate vital functions of his body from the inside out.

Principles of Chiropractic

There are many principles which mold the chiropractic philosophy, but perhaps the most pivotal and major principle is that a universal intelligence exists in all matter, including the human body, which continually gives organized matter its properties and actions, thus maintaining its existence.

Another key principle of the chiropractic philosophy is that good health is the expression of innate, or naturally existing, intelligence functioning through an inborn guiding and healing life energy. When transmission of this life energy is interrupted by barriers, such as misaligned spinal vertebrae impinging the nerves of the spinal column, the result is a decrease in the body's ability to heal and regulate itself.

The philosophy of chiropractic medicine plays an ongoing and integral part of what today has become a wellness revolution; a philosophy whose principles embrace the knowledge that the human body is designed to function as a whole, not as a collection of isolated parts. As such, chiropractic holds great promise in the struggle to reign in not only back pain, but even the debilitating effects of diabetes, sciatica, arthritis, seizures, and a myriad of other disorders through drug-free, non-invasive, natural treatment.

As a science, chiropractic addresses the relationship between the spine and the central nervous system, as well as this relationship's effect on the body's innate ability to heal itself and maintain good health. So, while chiropractic treatment does not *heal* your body, it does restore your body's inborn ability to heal itself.

As an art, chiropractic utilizes over a century of knowledge, combined with skill and dexterity to locate and correct vertebral misalignments that can impair the body's innate ability to maintain the good health we were born to enjoy.

The Energy of Life:
Our Connection to The Universe

When studying the chiropractic philosophy, you will likely come across the terms "universal intelligence", "innate intelligence", "innate energy", and "quantum healing." These principles are truly the cornerstones of chiropractic, and topics that are not only fascinating but also worthy of a deeper understanding.

Universal Intelligence

The primary principle of chiropractic is universal intelligence. Put simply, universal intelligence is the basic belief that nothing in the natural order of the universe is random; the belief that our existence is not a matter of mere luck.

Universal intelligence is not necessarily a religious or spiritual belief. While many people do believe that God is the source of universal intelligence, many others accept the concept of a universal intelligence outside the parameters of religion. They simply accept that some sort of intelligence must exist in order to create and propagate the myriad of glorious creatures and plants which inhabit our world.

Think about universal intelligence this way. Is it pure dumb luck that a bird's wing is aerodynamically perfect for flight? Or that fish have the ability to breathe underwater, but not on dry ground? What about a plant knowing that its roots must go down into the earth in order to sustain itself with water and nutrients, while its leaves must go up where sunshine and air are abundant? To think that these natural miracles just happen as a result of some random, chaotic accident is absurd.

Universal intelligence is rooted in logical, deductive reasoning. As one accepts and embraces the fact that the living things which inhabit the universe are *not* random collections of molecules created by chance and without any semblance of organization, the principle of universal intelligence becomes a point of deductive reasoning. And by deductive reasoning, one must reach the conclusion that this intelligence applies to every part of the universe, including the human body.

Innate Intelligence

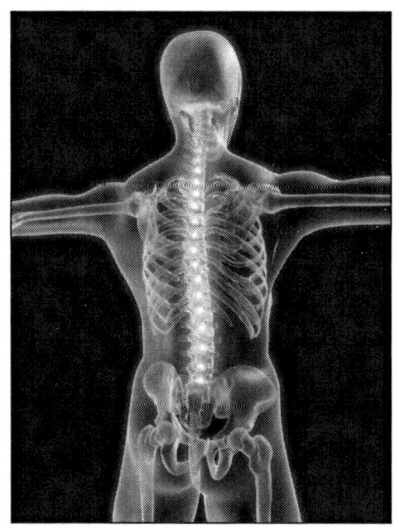

Acknowledging the existence of a universal intelligence dovetails directly into another basic principle of chiropractic philosophy – that of innate intelligence. Innate intelligence holds forth that in every living thing, be it plant, animal or human being, there is an inborn intelligence that constantly guides it on the path to a healthy existence.

Innate intelligence has nothing to do with education or the ability to learn. Rather, it speaks of the knowledge that every living thing is born with. It is this knowledge that allows plants and animals alike to adapt to their changing environment in order to thrive.

For example, have you ever placed a potted plant on a sunny windowsill? If so, you undoubtedly noticed that in a day or two, the majority of its leaves have turned to face the sun. That is an example of the plant's innate intelligence. The plant obviously does not have the ability to think or reason; it has no education to tell it that it must have sunshine in order to survive. Its inborn knowledge causes it to push its roots deep into the soil and keep its leaves above ground where they can absorb life-giving sunshine.

But what of human beings? How does innate intelligence play into our existence?

It is innate intelligence that tells our hearts how many times to beat every moment of every day, and how often we must fill our lungs with air in order to provide vital oxygen to our hearts. Innate intelligence tells our digestive system how to absorb nutrients from food and water and how to eliminate waste. Innate intelligence produces the anti-bodies to fight infection, cools our internal systems via perspiration, and tells us when our bodily structures require recuperative sleep. Innate intelligence is also the source of our self-preservation instinct, sometimes called the "fight or flight" response.

Doctors often admit that medical science has done all that it can possibly do for a sick or injured patient, and that the rest is up to the patient himself. What these health professionals are actually saying is that innate intelligence must now take over. If the body *can* be healed of its sickness or injury, the body will heal itself.

Innate Energy

Universal intelligence is repeated in all parts of the ordered universe both large and small, imparting both innate intelligence and innate energy into all living things.

Natural energy abounds throughout the universe, and many scientists embrace the theory that the universe was actually created by a massive burst of energy (the "big bang theory"). Whether you agree with this controversial theory or not, it is very evident that energy is constantly at work around us.

Consider the force that causes waves to crash ashore, wind to gust to hurricane force, and lightning to explode through the sky. These are all examples of innate energy. As thinking humans, we may learn how to harness the effects of this naturally occurring innate energy, but we will never be able to control the energy itself.

There is an order and intelligence to these forces of natural energy that are controlled by a universal intelligence. And this universal intelligence utilizes innate energy to perpetuate and maintain the existence of all living things. The very fact that the human body is an organized mass of molecules implies that humans, along with every other living being, are energetic entities.

For example, it is no coincidence that the human body runs on the innate energy of electricity. It is electricity that serves as the conduit for innate intelligence to keep the heart beating and respiratory system breathing, even when we are asleep or unconscious. Our innate intelligence adapts the universal force of electricity to sustain life and ensure survival.

The intelligence and energy that made the body can also heal the body. Vibrant good health does not come from medication, surgery or a doctor's education. It comes from the body's own innate intelligence to survive and rejuvenate.

Quantum Healing

According to Deepak Chopra, a leader in Ayurvedic medicine, quantum healing is this: "Quantum healing is healing the body and mind from a quantum level. That means from a level which is not manifested at a sensory level. Our bodies ultimately are fields of information, intelligence, and energy. Quantum healing involves a shift in the fields of energy information, so as to bring about a correction in an idea that has gone wrong. So quantum healing involves healing one mode of consciousness, the mind, to bring about changes in another mode of consciousness, the body."

Quantum healing embraces the belief that every thought, feeling, attitude, or instinct that you have affects your physical health on a cellular level. It takes the whole person into consideration, including mind, body, and soul. Quantum healing investigates what is being depleted within the body at a cellular level, and how the mind and spirit affect such an imbalance.

For example, quantum healing takes into consideration factors such as:

* ❖ Are you receiving enough nutrients and vitamins in your diet?
* ❖ Are you eating and resting properly?
* ❖ Are you carrying too much excess body weight?
* ❖ Are you happy?
* ❖ Are you getting enough physical exercise?
* ❖ Are you spending too much time alone?

The Cellular Biology of Innate Intelligence and Its Role in Quantum Healing

Our bodies are constructed of trillions of microscopic cells, and until recently it was widely believed that genetics, not environment, controlled these cells. However, recent scientific revelations have revealed that the environment and a cell's perception of that environment are what really control cellular behavior.

Signals such as temperature and light trigger signals inside a cell, prompting specific actions or reactions from within. And here's what is really fascinating … cellular perception is influenced by a person's beliefs, which goes back to the theory of quantum healing.

Memory patterns create beliefs, both conscious and unconscious, and most of our behaviors spring from these unconscious beliefs and expectations. The environment that surrounds a child early in life shapes the memory patterns, beliefs, and attitudes that person will carry into adulthood. So beliefs you do not even realize you have can, and most likely will, dramatically affect not only the choices you make in life, but also shape your physical wellbeing.

Quantum healing embraces the belief that the mind can, indeed, overcome cellular deficiencies and disease by removing the unseen barriers that interfere with innate healing. But the mind can also keep you shackled to sickness, depending on whether you control your thoughts and attitudes or they control you. So be aware and careful of your thoughts and attitudes, as well as the words you speak. Verbalizing thoughts, beliefs and attitudes, whether negative or positive, is an incredibly powerful process that can often directly affect your physical being.

The bottom line is this: your memory patterns do not have to define you or sentence you to an unhappy, unhealthy existence. However, it does take dedication and conviction to change negative thought patterns into positive ones. The choice to be happy and healthy is within your grasp.

Pain and Your Amazing Nervous System: The Nature and Purpose of Pain

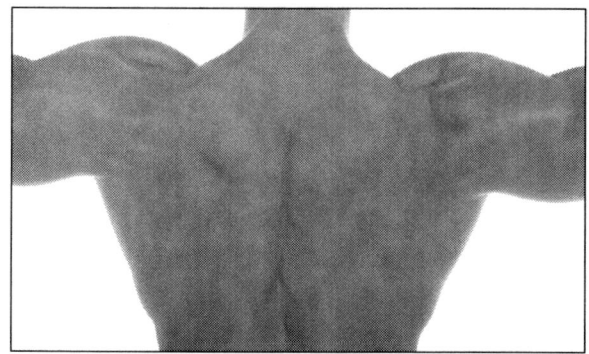

The nervous system is truly an extraordinary miracle of design. It controls every aspect of your body's functions, from tasting, smelling, seeing, hearing, thinking, running, sleeping, laughing, and speaking to feeling pain or pleasure. Literally every breath you take and every beat of your heart is governed by your nervous system.

How Nerves Work

The brain functions in your body as an incredibly powerful "computer mainframe." It not only stores a lifetime of memories, it also controls and coordinates the function of the billions of nerves that network throughout your body. These nerves, as just mentioned, control both the voluntary and involuntary functions of your body.

Some nerves have the function of sensation, while other nerves control muscle movement. Still other nerves reside deep within your body and work to keep your internal organs functioning properly.

So how does the brain communicate with all these billions of nerves? The spinal cord is an internal super information highway for the enormous network of nerves that threads throughout your entire body. Each one of these billions of nerves is constantly transmitting messages to the brain as well as receiving them. These lightning-fast messages contain a myriad of information from both the body's internal and external environments.

In order for these messages to be received by the brain, they must travel through the spinal cord.

Conversely, information and instructions from the brain to individual nerves travel through the spine to facilitate specific actions or movements. This constant two-way flow of information occurs in a matter of just milliseconds – twenty-four hours a day, every day of your life.

It is no wonder, then, that the human brain is considered a marvel of science, literally a "super computer" hidden deep inside your body, and that the spinal cord is called its "super information highway."

Anatomy of The Fragile Nervous System

Comprised of the brain, spinal cord, nerve roots, and peripheral nerves, the nervous system is not only incredibly complex, it is also amazingly fragile. In fact, the miniscule weight of one thin dime placed on a spinal nerve root will reduce that nerve root's ability to transmit signals by as much as 60%.

Think of it this way: If you step on a water hose or kink it in any way, the flow of water is considerably impaired. The same principle applies to nerve roots. Any type of mechanical pressure, such as a fall, automobile accident, or any other sort of trauma can have the effect of dramatically impairing the flow of information both going from and into the nerve. Even poor posture or a few extra pounds of body weight can adversely affect the nervous system.

The human nervous system is comprised of the central nervous system and the peripheral nervous system. The central nervous system is made up of the brain and spinal cord, and it controls the majority of your bodily functions. The peripheral nervous system is located just beyond the central nervous system, although they are connected to each other. The peripheral nervous system provides the supply of nerves to the rest of your body, relaying messages to and from the central nervous system.

It is the peripheral nervous system that sends a message of pain when you touch something hot or experience an injury of some sort. The central nervous system receives this pain message and transmits it to the brain. Incredibly, this entire pain/response impulse occurs in a split second, traveling at speeds up to 250 miles per hour.

The Problems and Gifts of Pain

The basic, primal purpose of pain is to warn you of impending injury or injury that has already occurred. For example, as mentioned above, touching something hot initiates a self-protection pain response. Pain is your body's built-in "alarm system," one that lets you know when something is has gone wrong with or is harming a bodily function.

Misaligned spinal vertebrae, compressed nerve roots or herniated spinal disks, as well as a number of other spinal disorders, can all result in pain. However, the source of the pain is not always easy to pinpoint. It can manifest as a migraine headache, shooting pain in the legs or arms, reduced range of motion, impaired vision or thought processes, or even high blood pressure, seizures, depression, digestive ailments, and the myriad of diseases associated with an impaired immune system.

Injury to a nerve, called neuropathic pain, can be horribly debilitating, and be relatively unresponsive to most conventional medical treatment such as painkillers or surgery.

It may sound odd, but in many ways, pain is also a gift. When your body sounds an alarm by generating a pain impulse, you have the opportunity to correct the situation either by ceasing the painful behavior or by seeking the care of a qualified health professional. Without such an alarm, a potentially harmful health condition can continue to degenerate until it is beyond repair.

Chiropractic Succeeds Where Other Pain Treatments Fail

In numerous studies, chiropractic has proven to be one of the most effective treatments for pain. However, the very foundation of chiropractic is not actually based upon the relief of pain. Pain relief is one of the wonderful side effects of a properly functioning spinal system, which includes the nervous system.

Rather than rely on chemical painkillers which have the potential to cause great harm, or an invasive surgery that presents an entirely different set of risks without any guarantee of relief, chiropractic doctors understand that health is the natural state of the physical body. This health is best maintained through supporting the body in a natural, non-invasive way. This is accomplished by restoring the body's natural functioning and eliminating obstacles or barriers which impede health and result in pain, instead of simply treating the symptoms caused by such obstacles.

Contrary to popular belief, chiropractic care addresses much more than musculoskeletal pain. In order to help people live healthier, fuller lives, it must also involve the care and maintenance of the nervous system.

This care is based upon the chiropractic philosophy that the same natural, innate intelligence capable of growing a single cell into a complex human being comprised of trillions of cells is also capable of healing and maintaining that same body if the nervous system is free of barriers or disturbances.

Helping You Help Yourself:
How Chiropractic Treatment Goes to the Source and Initiates Self-Healing

There are many ways to treat the symptoms of back pain but there are also several means to healing the problems that cause discomfort in the first place. For instance, traditional medical approaches such as medication work very well in alleviating symptoms of back pain. Also, hot and cold therapies provide an example of this type of treatment because they are beneficial in treating the inflammation and detoxifying the muscle; however, they do not address the problem that led to a strained, inflamed muscle in the first place.

Chiropractic treatment, on the other hand, addresses the complications that lead to back pain. Moreover, the chiropractic philosophy is based on restoring the body's natural functioning. Chiropractic specialists achieve this by focusing on the spinal mobility. Their mission is to manipulate the spine so that movement is no longer restricted. Since chiropractors believe that an imbalanced spine causes muscle spasms in the first place, they work to correct the problems and thus alleviate the back pain.

Furthermore, chiropractors perform an adjustment by applying a controlled, abrupt force to a joint. You may hear a cracking or popping sound but this is no cause for alarm. Many people think it is because bones are grinding together as the adjustment is made. Rather, it is simply the sound of the joint surfaces as they separate.

Moreover, it is also important to remember that chiropractors can manipulate the spine without making any sound at all. It all depends on your body and how it responds to this form of treatment. Of course, before this phase of the treatment begins, chiropractors usually incorporate passive physical therapy techniques such as ultrasound and Transcutaneous Electrical Nerve Stimulation (TENS). Some even use massage therapy to relax muscles before making adjustments.

Energy, Intelligence, and the Self-healing Body

What many patients do not know about chiropractic care is that its philosophies are centered on the innate intelligence of the human body. Innate intelligence, often referred to as universal intelligence, is characterized by the body's natural ability to govern itself.

The nervous system acts as a medium for the innate intelligence to communicate throughout the body. Most importantly, chiropractors believe that vertebral subluxations obstruct this communication; they strive to relieve the body of such interferences. The philosophy of chiropractic treatment is that many treatment options only alleviate back pain and, of course, that surgery should always be a last resort.

Similarly, quantum healing, often referred to as quantum touch, is based on the belief that the body is made to be self-healing. Still, this form of therapy works when a quantum touch practitioner combines breathing and body awareness exercises.

The practitioner is responsible for tapping into what is called life-force energy, Chi or Prana. Using his hands, the practitioner touches the disturbed area. By maintaining a high vibrational life-force field, the practitioner assists the natural healing process through resonance. Of course, everything has vibrations.

When two things vibrate at different frequencies, there is a natural tendency for the two to synchronize. Furthermore, the patient's independent functions synchronize with those of the practitioner. The high vibrations of the practitioner's life-force energy begin to work at the quantum or subatomic level of the body. Then, more obvious parts of the body are affected.

For example, quantum touch practitioner and author Richard Gordon documented a case during which practitioner Robert Rasmusson performed quantum touch on a woman with scoliosis. Within 20 minutes, her bones were two-thirds of the way realigned. Intriguingly, the bones were moving right before their eyes.

How Pain Can Help You Gain Good Health

Though most people have no desire to experience pain, it is a very important function of the human body. Sensations of pain alert us when something harmful is occurring in our bodies. From simple messages such as an object that is too hot to a more complex condition like sciatica (commonly referred to as a pinched nerve), pain, though undesirable, is important.

Of course, without nerves, these critical messages would not reach the brain. Most nerves connect to the central nervous system through the spinal cord. Afferent nerves, for instance, send messages *to* the central nervous system while efferent nerves transmit messages *from* the central nervous system to muscles and glands. Even though pain is an essential part of the body's communication to the brain, it can also be debilitating.

People with back pain, for example, are especially aware of how pain can adversely affect the quality of life. A conversation with a once-active pregnant woman whose back pain has become so unbearable she feels she can hardly move, or even a hard-working man who has such severe back pain he can barely sleep at night would indeed show that pain can hinder one's ability to function.

Moreover, this is where chiropractic treatment provides the solution for so many patients who are living with back pain. It is not enough just to treat the pain. The body builds a tolerance to many pain medications and many others adversely affect the gastrointestinal functions and even the cardiovascular system.

Passive therapies such as ultrasound and TENS treatments must be performed under the supervision of a licensed medical professional. Of course, the patient should not be expected to live with the pain outside the doctor's office. Fortunately, chiropractic treatment succeeds where other passive treatments fail.

After all, the only way to stop the pain is to provide a cure for its source. Whether you are interested in spinal manipulation or a more alternative treatment like quantum healing, you will find that chiropractic treatment allows your body to achieve healing in its own right and most often, for good.

The Road to Recovery Begins with Your Own Superhighway

When most people think of chiropractic treatment, they envision a practitioner adjusting the spine. They might imagine the cracking sound as the chiropractor confidently turns the patient's head. However, what most people do not know all that much about this form of therapy.

Most people are completely unaware that the central theme of chiropractic treatment is self healing. In fact, most practitioners who work with chiropractic treatment view themselves as facilitators; thus, they believe that they are making a way for the body to function normally by removing subluxations and re-establishing communication within the body. This concept seems surprising until you consider how the intricacy of the human body. More specifically, consider the spinal cord and its ever-important role as a means of communication.

The Body's Information Superhighway Should Be Free of Roadblocks

Though it may sound cliché, the spine and spinal cord really do serve as an information superhighway for the human body. Moreover, the nervous system uses this highway to direct traffic, delivering information from the brain to other areas of the body, and also retrieving messages and delivering them back to the brain.

As almost every driver will admit, there are very few occurrences more inconvenient than road construction. It often causes drivers to take a detour, which is typically congested and takes much longer than the normal route. Similar conditions exist in the spinal cord when it is obstructed by vertebral subluxations, which occur when one or more spinal vertebrae lose their proper positions with adjacent vertebrae. This complication interferes with nerves and thus hinders communication within the nervous system.

While this may not sound serious, vertebral subluxations must not be taken lightly or ignored. For example, vertebral subluxations can easily be compared to termites in a home. After all, termites move slowly but deliberately. The house may look normal on the outside but deep within its walls, it is gradually eroding. You have the choice of ignoring the termites or getting treatment to eradicate them. By the time the floor caves in, irreversible damage has occurred.

The same is true for the health of your spine. It is always best to address a problem when it begins. Back pain serves as an indicator that something is amiss. Disregarding it may only lead to future complications or a health problem that only continues to get worse.

Mechanism of Back Injury Is Often Slow and Deliberate

It is important to remember that many back injuries are not sudden, highly traumatic episodes. Instead, they are brought on by the everyday stresses the body endures. For instance, the UPS employee who spends his entire workday loading and unloading packages from trucks is a candidate for back injury because he places slow, continuous stress on his spine.

Eventually, he will lift a heavier package, one that would not normally pose a problem for him. But that last heavy package after a long workday of lifting is likely to damage his fatigued muscles. That leaves chiropractic specialists to conclude that the mechanism of injury was not the heavy package (which, again, would not normally be too heavy), but the repetitive lifting that caused harm to the patient.

The mechanism of injury is best defined by Brian Dale, a certified emergency dispatch instructor and Chief of the Salt Lake City Fire Department. In his article titled, "The Energy Within: Mechanism of Injury and the EMD," he defines mechanism of injury as, "the exchange of forces that results in injury to the patient(s)." Of course, Mr. Dale is speaking in terms of an auto accident.

He goes on to say that the force from the automobile and the object it struck leads to the injury. However, he also mentions that the force does not stop at the place of impact. Rather, organs within the body collide as a result of the impact. This type of reasoning can certainly be applied to the UPS employee. The mechanism of injury here begins with the repetitive lifting and ends with the force of the last heavy package, which strains the fatigued muscles and forces the worker to stop his activity. Moreover, the pain finally compels him to address the complications that are causing pain in the first place.

Relief of Nerve Pressure Means Freedom to Resume Normal Activities

Fortunately, the UPS employee does not have to entertain the possibility of a career change in order to find pain relief. Instead, there are adjustments that should be made. While there are proactive approaches to preventing future back pain (back braces, muscle strengthening and conditioning exercises, etc), chiropractic treatment is the only passive therapy that offers fast relief that addresses the cause of back pain and does not just alleviate its symptoms.

Of course, some patients are wary of seeking this form of therapy because they do not completely understand how it works. However, the process is actually quite simple. You should not allow intimidation to stand between you and pain relief. Following is some information about how chiropractic treatment relieves nerve pressure and removes road blocks from your information superhighway.

First, chiropractic treatment begins with an examination of the entire spine. When a chiropractor finds a subluxation, he addresses it by making a spinal adjustment to that specific area. An adjustment simply places the joint back into its normal position. Finally, it reintroduces motion to the stiffened joint and flushes fluid from the irritated area. Additionally, the adjustment opens the space in between the joints where nerves normally travel. Thus, the road block is no longer able to displace nerves and adversely affect the nervous system.

Most importantly, your treatment plan is based on your needs. There are many different chiropractic techniques that can be used to relieve interference, alleviate back pain, and help you lead a happy, healthy life. Here are a few of the most popular among many affective techniques offered by chiropractors.

Spinal Manipulation

Among the most popular technique is spinal manipulation. It is achieved through sudden, quick pressure applied to the spine, usually by hand or through turning. A popping or cracking sound may result but you should not be alarmed. This is simply caused by space opening up between the joints and gases such as nitrogen, oxygen, and carbon dioxide being released from the joint.

Sacro Occipital Technique (SOT)

"Sacro" refers to the sacrum, which is the foundation for the spine. Most people think of it as their tail bone. Furthermore, "Occipital" refers to the occiput, which is basically the back of the head. The goal of using SOT is to facilitate a stable between the bottom and top of the spine because this relationship has a profound affect on how the brain and spinal cord function.

Moreover, it combines chiropractic adjustments to the spine, visceral manipulation, cranial manipulation, extremity manipulation, and other work involving the muscles and ligaments. As previously discussed, adjustments relieve nerve pressure and thus correct subluxations. However, this is not always enough, when other manipulation treatments are incorporated as needed by the patient.

Flexion-Distraction Technique

This is the most widely used technique when it comes to treating disc injuries that cause back pain and even accompanying leg pain. It involves the use of a specialized table that gently distracts or stretches the spine, allowing the chiropractor to isolate the area of disc involvement and still flex the rest of the spine. This moves the disc away from the nerve; inflammation is reduced and pain in the back and leg is alleviated. Like most chiropractic treatments, flexion-distraction is applied in a series of treatments and is most often combined with home exercises.

Pelvic Blocking Techniques

During this a pelvic blocking treatment, the chiropractor places cushioned wedges under each side of the patient's pelvis. Combined with gentle maneuvers, draws the disc away from the nerve. Again, this technique is applied in a series of treatments and your condition is continuously monitored.

The most important point to remember is that there are a variety of chiropractic techniques available. Moreover, most practitioners are more than happy to customize a treatment plan that puts you on the road to recovery and allows your body to harness its self-healing ability.

Introduction to the
Mind-Body Connection

Just as chronic pain can have a profound effect on your emotions, the way you think and deal with emotion have direct effects on your physical wellbeing. Of course, there are health issues over which you have no control. You may become injured or challenged by a disease that just happened, not because you did something to make it happen.

When facing disease, many patients are confused because they led healthy lifestyles before their unfortunate diagnosis. Their response to the diagnosis may sound something like, "I've always been an active person. I watch my diet and I take supplements everyday. I take care of my body. I don't understand why this is happening to me."

The simple fact is that even healthy people face injury or disease at a given time. As difficult as it may be, it is crucial to take personal responsibility for your health. This includes taking care of the physical aspects when it comes to treating a condition, which means compliance with all treatments prescribed by your physician or specialist.

For example, if you have chronic back pain and your physician recommends a conditioning program with aerobic exercise three times per week, attend all three sessions each week, even if you are sore the first few times or simply have other things you would rather be doing. Following the doctor's orders not only keeps you physically healthy, it helps you to take control of your condition. In this way, you benefit on equally important levels, emotionally and mentally.

Personal responsibility for healthfulness includes not only physical maintenance but also careful attention to emotions, mental outlook, and how they are allowed to influence your health. In fact, the mind can have such a powerful influence over physical health that physicians like Dr. John E. Sarno believe that emotional and mental instability cause a condition called tension myositis syndrome (TMS).

Dr. Sarno believes that the mind chooses not to confront emotional stresses such as anxiety and anger. Instead, it represses these emotions to the unconscious by distracting itself with physical pain. This brain achieves this by decreasing blood flow to the muscles, typically those in the back, neck, shoulders, and buttocks. Moreover, decreased blood flow deprives the muscles of oxygen and causes pain.

Though the oxygen deprivation is mild, the pain can be fairly debilitating. Furthermore, the pain experienced by a person with TMS is real pain. The only difference between pain rooted in TMS and pain from a physical ailment is that its true cause is mental rather than physical. For instance, most back pain is caused by strained muscles or pressure on nerve roots along the spinal column. In contrast, pain from TMS is caused by repressed mental anxiety. Meanwhile, decreased blood flow and oxygen deprivation are merely symptoms of the real problem. Hence, TMS provides a perfect example of how a patient's emotional and mental wellbeing can affect health, even back and neck pain.

Moreover, physicians like Dr. Sarno refer to this phenomenon as the mind-body connection, which basically refers to how mental and emotional states affect a patient's physical being. Just as there are treatments to heal physical injuries, there are also techniques which patients can use to make the mind-body connection work toward their healing.

In order to treat TMS, the patient must address the mental issues that trigger it. After receiving a physical exam to ensure that there are no physical injuries, the next step is to focus on the anxiety and anger the brain is working so hard to repress. One way to achieve this is to keep a journal documenting the source or sources of the emotional distress.

For example, traumatic life events such as child abuse, divorce, or death of a loved one might incite anger or anxiety. Moreover, personality type is also said to trigger these emotions, particularly if the person is a perfectionist of sorts, experiences guilt easily, or is self-critical. Nevertheless, the key to overcoming TMS is to repetitively document these traumatic events or personality characteristics in order to form a correlation between these situations and the pain they are causing. As the mind begins to grasp what is actually occurring, it stops trying to deceive itself. Of course, journaling is only one way to make the connection between mind and body. There are several more techniques. Here is a brief overview:

Biofeedback

This process monitors a patient's heart rate, blood pressure, and even muscle tension with electronic monitoring devices. Once the patient is made aware of these biological changes, she has a better understanding of why they occur and how to regulate them.

Guided Imagery

This technique uses the patient's imagination to promote relaxation and healing of a particular illness. For example, when a pregnant woman is past her due date, some midwives and doulas recommend that she imagine her cervix dilating. This imagery is so strong that women have reported they went into labor within hours of practicing it.

Hypnotherapy

During hypnotherapy, the patient is guided into a deep state of relaxation. She is directed to certain images provided by the therapist and hypnosis allows the patient to become completely engaged in them. They may vary depending on the condition needing treatment. Furthermore, hypnotherapy has been shown to aid in weight loss and help patients quit smoking.

Meditation

Though meditation is often practiced from a spiritual perspective, it is also effective from a medical point of view. In a religious context, meditation is designed to facilitate spiritual growth. However, regardless of religious or cultural background, all patients can benefit from this technique. It is beneficial because it assists in deep relaxation, which helps to alleviate the stress and anxiety that are so often the true causes of back pain.

Why You Should Be Conscious of the Unconscious Mind

Though most people devote very little conscious thought to their unconscious mind, it can have a profound effect on behaviors and health. When dealing with back pain, your mental outlook has a tremendous affect on the amount of pain you feel as well as how well you recover. While you may not consciously desire to live with pain, your unconscious mind may be telling you that there is no other option.

Of course, this raises the question of how to access this mysterious part of the mind and chance the misconceptions that lead to unnecessary pain. Nevertheless, in order to utilize the unconscious mind, it is important to understand how it functions, influences your thought process, and affects behavior.

How The Unconscious Mind Works

First of all, the unconscious mind can be discussed in two distinct parts, the subconscious and the superconscious. The subconscious retains everything ranging from childhood experiences to the daily occurrences of a person's life. This includes genetic, social, and religious experiences, whether they were big events which had a tremendous impact or the small, less memorable activities of daily life.

The subconscious simply retains all this information indiscriminately, rejecting none of it. Since the conscious mind analyzes this information, it can only retain so much at a given time. Thus, its overflow moves to the subconscious, which is designed to store information rather than analyze it. Meanwhile, the super-conscious is best described as part of the spiritual realm of a person's mind. Although people are largely unaware of its influence, the unconscious mind plays a major role in how people behave, even when it comes to their health.

For example, many weight-loss specialists agree that the unconscious mind can cause people to compulsively overeat. They believe that the impulse to eat for comfort begins at infancy. When an infant cries, his or her mother offers him or her nice warm milk. In most cases, this provides comfort and tranquility to the child. Sometimes, the infant may not even be hungry.

Moreover, people do not consciously remember being nursed to sleep in the warm arms of their caretakers, but their unconscious mind does remember. Thus, it still correlates food with comfort. As another example, think of a person who has repeatedly injured his back. Perhaps he has tried several treatment options in order to alleviate the pain with no results. Eventually, this patient will subconsciously believe there is no cure in sight. Though further attempts might be made, the unconscious mind will associate treatment with failure. Of course, this fundamentally unknown aspect of the human mind affects not only behavior but also self-image.

Automatic Thoughts Can Be Convincing

It may seem cliché or just overly negative to say that the world is a cruel place to exist, but this is true some of the time. Everyone encounters negativity during various times in his life. Unfortunately, some are challenged by it more than others. Some people do not know how to deal with these negative messages. Thus, the messages remain in the unconscious mind, which indiscriminately accepts them.

Not knowing why feelings of anxiety or self-doubt exist, a person might try to consciously reverse these feelings by repeating positive affirmations to his or herself. While this is a good thought, that is all it will ever be. For example, a man on his way to a job interview may be assuring himself by saying, "I have a lot to offer this company. I am ready for this interview." However, if his unconscious mind is convinced, "I am terrible at job interviews," the positive thoughts will only be discarded.

The main problem with thoughts from the unconscious mind is that they are automatic. In contrast, thoughts from the conscious mind are analyzed and deliberate. Going back to the job interview example, the man who was reassuring himself was making a conscious effort, choosing the right words, and making a genuine attempt to reassure himself.

However, the nagging thought about being terrible during job interviews was automatic. As for the patient with back pain, those thoughts may run in this sequence: The patient consciously thinks, "This is it. I know this is going to work. I know several other people who used it and they feel much better." In spite of this, the unconscious mind maintains, "Nothing ever works for me." Automatic thoughts come to mind so quickly that they can almost be thought of as a mental reflex. Though the situation may seem hopeless, it is essential to identify negative thoughts from the unconscious mind. Once this is achieved, you are already making progress toward recovery.

The Next Step Is to Take Control

From this point, it becomes your responsibility to take control of your thoughts and emotions. In some situations, the cause of a patient's back pain is physical. Still, his or her mental outlook has a significant effect on how well the healing process progresses. For other patients, their mental outlook alone may be the root of their back pain. In either case, there are steps you can take to counteract negative thoughts. Even thoughts originating deep within the unconscious mind do not have to be a hindrance any longer.

Automatic Thoughts Can Be Used to Your Advantage

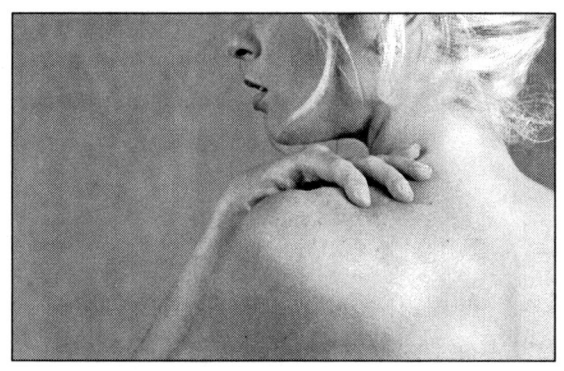

The unconscious mind becomes a pool of information taken along throughout a person's entire life. These thoughts, both positive and negative, are stored away. Though they continue to affect your attitude, behavior, and even your health, you are most likely unaware of them. Furthermore, if you received the same information repeatedly, it becomes embedded into the unconscious mind.

It is very much a part of who you are. Thus, information stored in the unconscious mind is likely to surface in the form of automatic thoughts. Of course, these thoughts can be both positive and negative; however, negative thinking may adversely affect your health or even cause pain. Fortunately, you do not have to live with negative thinking or allow it to influence your health. There are many ways to combat negativity and inspire your mind to improve your wellbeing, not impair it.

The Art of Positive Thinking

In some situations, thinking positive takes effort. A person facing chronic back pain, for example, may find it difficult to stay positive through the pain, especially if he has attempted several different treatment options unsuccessfully. Still, even in this situation, utilizing the art of positive thinking is possible. In fact, there are several easy ways to integrate affirmative thoughts into your day.

These affirmative statements will begin to combat the negativity, eliminating it from your life. For instance, begin by deciding what it is you would like to achieve. Imagine that your goal is to find relief from lower back pain. You would begin by making a positive, concise statement such as, "I would like for my lower back to get stronger and feel better."

Moreover, it is important to remember that your mind is highly visual and thinks in pictures. Accordingly, an appropriate mental image might be you working out on an elliptical machine and going past your usual time, or spending more time at your aqua aerobics class because your strength has improved. Also, combine these mental images with an affirmative thought such as, "My lower back is stronger and stronger each day."

It is also essential to use only positive words and avoid words like "not." For example, an inappropriate statement would be, "I do not feel any pain today." For one thing, there is a good chance you still feel some pain. Additionally, the word "not" evokes a negative image which would actually cause you to visualize yourself still in pain. If spoken words are not always enough, some patients write positive statements on notes and strategically place the notes where they will find them later. Some examples of good places to leave notes may be your gym bag, medicine cabinet, or kitchen silverware drawer.

Going Against Negative Thoughts

While positive affirmation is crucial, there is more to the art of positive thinking. In order to replace the pessimism and improve your mental and physical wellbeing, you must identify and resist your natural tendencies to think negative. Furthermore, there are several themes that appear among these pessimistic thoughts.

First of all, negative thinkers tend to make extreme statements and judgments. They often over-generalize, judge people and things in the world around them, jump to conclusions about what others think of them, enlarge difficulties, and minimize positives. For example, a person with one or more of these tendencies may make a statement such as, "My back pain is never going to get better" or "She thinks my pain is made up." Not only does this thought process trigger mental illnesses like depression, it also affects back pain.

Because people who are judgmental toward others often judge themselves more severely, they actually incite their own anxiety. They make assumptions about what others think, usually assuming the worst. They are also quick to compare their situation with someone else's in a highly competitive way. This may work fine so long as the other person does not "win." However, if this competitor is unable to assume her place in the limelight, she is likely to feel like a failure.

Of course, there are simple ways to resist these negative, extreme thoughts. For instance, if you encounter one of these thoughts, simply apply logic. Write the thought down on paper and try to provide evidence in support of it. More than likely, there will be no evidence you can actually prove. Instead, you will find over-generalized, extreme, and judgmental statements you cannot prove. Working through this will help you identify negative thinking, allowing you to consciously go against it.

And finally, remember that changing something as complex as your thought process takes time and self-discipline. Even if it begins to feel redundant, continue to thwart negativity, and positively affirm what you expect to get out of your treatment. Moreover, even when the pessimistic thoughts continue to mock you, keep identifying and re-affirming the positive. You are making more of a difference than you realize. As a matter of fact, chronic pain and depression go hand-in-hand at times. Allowing your mind to revert to negativity could have a damaging effect on your health.

It All Starts in Your Head: Simple Techniques to Help You Change Your Thoughts

Chronic physical pain has the capacity to bring on far more than just physical discomfort. Patients with chronic back pain, for instance, are very susceptible to depression. This is especially true when the pain forces them to accept limitations. Back pain that prevents patients from assuming their normal everyday activity for an extended period of time leaves them vulnerable to feelings of hopelessness and defeat.

Likewise, feelings of anger, anxiety, and envy actually cause physical pain in some individuals. In many cases, these emotions become repressed because the brain actually initiates muscle pain in order to distract itself from the upsetting emotions. As previously discussed, one mechanism found in some patients occurs when the brain restricts blood flow to muscles in the back, neck, shoulders, and extremities. This causes a lack of oxygenation and thus triggers muscle pain.

Moreover, negative thinking which usually originates in the unconscious mind can make existing pain even worse. Even if the patient sustained an injury to a muscle or nerve, the way that individual responds mentally has a tremendous impact on the recovery process. Furthermore, negative thoughts will create a vicious cycle of back pain if left unchecked.

Fortunately, you do not have to live with a physically abusive unconscious mind. Rather, you can train your mind to think more positively. You can harness the same power that causes pain and use it for healing. One of the most difficult aspects of negative thinking is that it occurs automatically. No conscious thought is necessary for the mind to revert back to its unconscious negativity. This can make it difficult to identify pessimistic thinking and where it originates. Fortunately, there are a few thought processes that are common among patients with anxiety.

Extreme Thinking

People who practice extreme thinking are inclined to view life like a purely black and white photo. As you can imagine, this is not a pretty picture. Extreme thinkers see no grey and thus give themselves no room for mistakes or human shortcomings. Moreover, this affects not only their self-image but also how they see the world and all the other people living in it. When it comes to back pain, they become easily frustrated. If they are not completely pain-free, they are completely unsatisfied. Unfortunately, there are several types of back pain that can only be managed, not cured.

Sweeping Statements

While the thought process behind this is similar to extreme thinking, the words a patient speaks are the most damaging. For example, the person might say something like, "I'll never get better," or "this is the worst pain in the world." If sweeping statements like these are made often enough, they can severely inhibit a person's ability to recover from back pain. Such exaggerated speech makes it too easy for a patient to become caught up in the viscous circle of pain causing depression and more pain.

Making Judgments and Assumptions

These individuals tend to act as mind readers, often making assumptions about how others see them. Moreover, they are very judgmental when it comes to their own shortcomings and it spills over into their perception of other people. Thus, not only are judgers and assumers hard on themselves, they think that others are equally as unforgiving when it comes to their shortfalls. Not surprisingly, this can produce debilitating anxiety, anger, and frustration.

Keeping Up with the Jones Family

This condition is far more than just a cliché. It has far-reaching consequences and even physical pain. People who compare themselves and their lives to others' usually practice this in every area of their lives. This includes the cars they drive, the homes in which they live, their talents and, yes, even their health. In some situations, they triumph over the other person and enjoy a place in the spotlight. However, if they fall short, it can have a devastating effect on their mental wellbeing. As you can imagine, this is the source of anxiety for many people.

Larger Than Life Challenges

Some patients magnify their problems and minimize the solutions. By focusing on the challenges, they become consumed by them and see no way out. Family and friends may attempt to offer emotional support but every encouraging thought will be counteracted. Every treatment option seems as though it simply will not be enough to heal the terrible pain. This mentality allows a patient to give up hope and slip into anxiety and depression.

So What?

The common setback in each of these situations is the lack of reasonable thinking. After all, statements like, "I'll never feel better" do not make any sense. Thus, when faced with negative thoughts like these, ask yourself if it makes sense to have these feelings or make such radical statements. Once you recognize the automatic thought, take action against it next time when it resurfaces. Many people interrupt the thought by asking, "So what?" For instance, when a thought comes to mind and says, "My back hurts. It will never go away." Simply ask, "So what? So what if it doesn't? My doctor and I will find a way to manage it."

Asking this simple question can be a significant step in breaking the vicious cycle of back pain and anxiety. After all, just as it is important to follow the prescribed treatments when dealing with physical pain, it is equally crucial to take steps in improving mental health. Eliminating negative thinking prevents the mind from causing the body pain and helps existing physical pain become manageable.

The Relaxation Response: A Technique That Utilizes The Power of Belief

When most people imagine what it means to relax, they might dream of a tropical vacation or simply a favorite book and a warm cup of coffee. While such activities may be very enjoyable, they do not encourage true relaxation. Furthermore, people are bombarded with messages about how unhealthy society has become. If this is not stressful enough, their minds are overrun by different opinions of how to stay healthy and protect their families.

Of course, this stress is in addition to the everyday stresses that relationships, family life, and work may bring. Naturally, it is very difficult for people to truly relax. There are breakthrough techniques that tap into the mind-body connection and help people achieve genuine, fulfilling relaxation. This is not limited to a beach scene with a cold beverage and a little pink umbrella. This form of relaxation has the power to encourage healing.

A Few Simple Steps to Physical Wellbeing

Reaching a state of true relaxation is not difficult. In fact, Dr. Herbert Benson designed a relaxation technique called the Relaxation Response that takes only two steps. First, Dr. Benson asks the patient to choose a prayer, word, sound or muscular activity to repeat. The words can be spiritually inspiring or secular. The most important point to remember is that the word, sound, or motion should help the person feel calm and peaceful. Second, when everyday thoughts inhibit concentration, simply focus on the repetition and ignore distractions.

Additionally, these two simple steps can be broken down into six more specific steps. You may find this helpful if you have no previous experience with relaxation or meditation techniques.

- ❖ First, begin by sitting in a comfortable position and closing your eyes.

- ❖ Then, relax all of your muscles beginning with your feet and progressing upward until you have relaxed the muscles in your face.

- ❖ Next, be sure to pay close attention to your breathing. You should breathe naturally; although, some therapists who recommend this technique tell their patients to inhale and exhale through their noses.

- ❖ Maintain a positive attitude. When your mind begins to doubt how well you are practicing the technique, tell yourself, "Oh, well." Just brush the doubt aside and focus on your breathing as well as the repetition of your chosen word.

❖ Depending on your schedule, you may continue for 10 to 20 minutes before getting up. Of course, you should not stand up right away. Instead, remain sitting for awhile and allow some thoughts to come back into your conscious mind. And lastly, this technique should be performed once or twice daily for the best results.

Most importantly, keep in mind that this technique is far more than just relaxing. It eliminates anxiety and allows the mind to focus on healing. After all, the mind-body connection has proven itself powerful in many situations. In fact, just as physical pain can trigger depression and anxiety, unhealthy attitudes can actually cause physical pain. Moreover, Dr. Benson takes this principle a step further.

The Power of Belief

While many physicians disregard the placebo effect, Dr. Benson believes that it is the answer for many patients facing various health issues, especially those dealing with any form of pain. When testing new medications, researchers rely on placebo pills to measure the effectiveness of new drugs. In many cases, patients noticed physical changes even while taking placebos.

Placebo pills contain inert ingredients, indicating the physical changes were a result of mental attitude. Rather than ignoring mental attitude, Dr. Benson believes patients should use it to promote healing. Thus, implementing a relaxation technique allows patients to mentally focus on healing the pain, pushing aside any doubt and believing in the healing they hope to achieve.

Furthermore, Dr. Benson has asserted that deep relaxation often becomes a spiritual experience and that the spiritual aspects enhance healing. During an interview cited by imagery4relaxation.com, Dr. Benson said,

"Belief can be translated into physical reality in the body. Belief can be translated into physical reality in the body. One can turn on a whole host of symptoms and diseases by simply believing them, and similarly they can be relieved. There is a whole list of diseases where belief has been shown to play a major role and it's a remarkable list, angina, asthma, all forms of pain, skin rashes, duodenal ulcers, rheumatoid arthritis, congestive heart failure, and on and on. One could even die because of belief."

Also, when asked how faith contributes to the power of health beliefs, Dr. Benson explained that people experience sp7irituality when they feel that a power, force, or energy is close to them and providing guidance. For most people, these two ingredients compose a spiritual experience. He also explained that 95 percent of all Americans believe in God and hold that as their most powerful belief.

For them, their strongest belief is in something beyond themselves. Therefore, since beliefs have the power to physically impact the health of a person's body, he or she should rely on the strongest belief. For most people, it is spiritual but some people choose to rely on secular beliefs. The most important factor is to truly believe that you will experience pain relief as a result of this technique. Moreover, Dr. Benson maintains that it should be like taking penicillin. You take the medication and expect results.

Eliciting the Relaxation Response

Once the Relaxation Response has been achieved, a person has tapped into his or her ability to promote physical healing and wellness through the mind. Of course, for some, eliciting the Relaxation Response may seem intimidating or even difficult. After all, the world has become a busy place and people's lives are increasingly hectic. Accomplishing such deep relaxation may seem next to impossible under the circumstances. Opportunely, there are several techniques patients can use to trigger deep relaxation and attain the healing and pain relief they need and deserve.

Relaxation Is a Breath Away

If you were to ask a woman who has experienced childbirth, she would most likely verify the importance of proper breathing exercises for both pain management and relaxation. Furthermore, breathing techniques can be implemented to help patients cope with all kinds of different muscle pain in addition to helping them achieve deep relaxation. In fact, most therapists agree that proper breathing is of paramount importance. Of course, breathing is an involuntary function; most patients have a tendency to take it for granted, assuming that they will be able to implement proper breathing. However, there are a few important points to remember about applying the correct breathing exercises to any relaxation technique.

Chest Breathing Versus Abdominal Breathing

For many people, most if not all breathing becomes restricted to the chest, which can lead to mild oxygen deprivation of the muscles. This is due to the fact that more of the blood flow takes place in the lower lobes of a person's lungs. Chest breathers do not fully expand the lower lobes, which translates to decreased oxygen transfer in the blood. Of course, chest breathers are usually people who experience chronic stress, which leads to short, shallow breathing in the first place.

In contrast, abdominal breathing, also called diaphragmatic breathing, offers many benefits. Among these, it improves the circulation of blood and lymph. Moreover, lymph is rich with immune cells and helps prevent infection. Most importantly, abdominal breathing promotes the Relaxation Response.

How to Practice Abdominal Breathing

Fortunately, there are steps you can take to implement abdominal breathing as part of your relaxation technique.

- ❖ Begin by placing your right hand over your chest and your left hand over your abdomen.

- ❖ Take a breath as you would naturally and watch how your hands rise. The left hand should rise before the right hand. This means you are filling up the lower areas of the lungs first, which provides for optimal circulation.

- ❖ Next, take a deep breath, inhaling deeply through your nose. Hold the breath for seven seconds or less, whatever feels most comfortable. Of course, it is highly recommended that you do not exceed seven seconds.

- ❖ Then, exhale through your mouth, emptying all remaining air from the lungs. By contracting the abdominal muscles, you can be sure the air is forced from the lungs completely. Emptying the lungs of remaining air helps to ensure deeper breathing. Also, it is important to remember that exhaling should last twice as long as inhaling. Many patients find it helpful to count as they breathe in and out.

- ❖ And finally, you may repeat the abdominal breathing exercise until you become completely acquainted with it.

Abdominal Breathing and the Relaxation Response

When you are comfortable with abdominal breathing and ready to use it as a relaxation technique, you may also add one or more of the other methods. Of course, there are several ways to elicit the relaxation response. Many people implement a combination of progressive muscle relaxation (usually beginning with the feet and moving upward), repetition of words, sounds or prayers, meditation, guided imagery, and even exercise programs like yoga or tai chi. As you may already notice, abdominal breathing is the easiest of these methods. Furthermore, it can be practiced anywhere with little effort.

The Anchoring Technique and How You Can Relax on Cue

Anchoring is a neurological response that occurs when the brain associates a memory or state change with a certain stimulus. For example you can choose a particular word, sound, prayer, or even a motion to act as your cue to relax. Many people practice this technique in combination with other relaxation exercises in order to trigger the Relaxation Response.

Moreover, repeating this word or phrase throughout your relaxation exercise, you are teaching the mind to associate this word with relaxation. After several sessions during which the anchoring technique is utilized, your mind will perceive the word as a verbal cue. Once you say it, your mind will automatically begin to unwind. Of course, it is essential that practice the anchoring technique only one or twice a day when you are eliciting the relaxation response. If you attempt to use the cue too often, you risk becoming desensitized to it.

Breathing Techniques Combined with Imagery Techniques

In essence, the brain thinks in pictures; thus, mental images are very important and even useful in creating a relaxing atmosphere. Because images are powerful and have the capacity to evoke an emotional response, it only makes sense that the proper images can facilitate relaxation.

Furthermore, imagery techniques can be used in combination with breathing techniques in order to initiate the relaxation response. For example, you may think of your garden as a peaceful, relaxing place. Thus, you can imagine yourself sitting quietly in the garden taking in deep breathes of fresh air. Of course, imagery is not limited to scenes. In fact, some patients prefer to visualize their "stress" as an object that can be folded away and locked in a safe or chest.

Picture Yourself Healthy

Imagery or visualization techniques are very beneficial and are used as an alternative treatment for various physical conditions. It has been proven as an effective way to facilitate self-healing for a variety of illnesses ranging from canker sores to cancer.

For example, researchers at Pennsylvania State University studied seven students who suffered from recurrent canker sores. They were instructed to imagine that their canker sores were being bathed in white blood cells. After beginning the visualization techniques, the students reported a significant decrease in canker sore outbreaks.

Additionally, a study conducted by researchers from Ohio State University found that cancer patients can also use visualization techniques beneficially in combination with chemotherapy. The study showed that patients who practiced relaxation techniques using imagery were more relaxed and better prepared about their therapy. Most importantly, they reported a more positive outlook than those who underwent treatment without using imagery techniques.

For instance, many cancer patients are asked to imagine that their bone marrow is steadily releasing white blood cells into the blood stream. If cells are too difficult to visualize, some patients picture their healthy cells as plump, ripe berries. Also, they imagine that the cancer cells are dried, withered fruit.

Meanwhile, the patient envisions his immune system as a flock of birds swooping in to carry away the withered fruit. Most importantly, many patients who perform these imagery techniques report that their white counts double by the time they go in for the next checkup.

Of course, those who advocate visualization techniques assert that one of the most important aspects of any self-healing technique is the patient's belief in it. One form of self-healing therapy is the utilization of the relaxation response, which was pioneered by Dr. Herbert Benson.

Furthermore, the Relaxation Response is achieved when the mind and body are in deep relaxation. This facilitates the mind-body connection to healing. Additionally, the Relaxation Response can be used to promote mental health by relieving anxiety, as well as promote physical health by allowing the patient to focus the body's energy on healing. Thus, you should think of these techniques in the same way you think of traditional medicine.

For example, when a physician prescribes a medication, especially something simple and straightforward like an antibiotic, most people take the medication and expect results. Therefore, you should have the same expectations when exercising any relaxation technique, whether it is visualization, word repetition, etc.

Moreover, there are several popular visualization techniques referred to as guided imagery because they require the assistance of a therapist. In addition, they are used not only for relaxation but also motivation; for example, motivational uses include cessation of smoking or accomplishment of weight loss goals.

Guided Waking Imagery

First, the patient is taught to envision a series of different settings. These might include a beach, pasture, mountain, house, and/or a swamp. Later, the patient's thoughts are analyzed by the therapist for sources of anxiety, conflict, illogical beliefs, and interpersonal problems.

In many cases, the emotions that cause anxiety are repressed to the unconscious mind. Unfortunately, they are not rendered dormant. Instead, they often lead to depression or even physical ailments such as sore muscles in the back, neck, shoulders, legs and arms. Identifying these repressed emotions is the often the first step to dealing with the true underlying cause of physical pain.

Autogenic Abreactions

This visualization technique is typically used to release the stresses of unpleasant life events that have been repressed, causing the patient to experience unhealthy anxiety. During this technique, a therapist asks the patient to practice passive acceptance toward his mental experiences. In this condition, the patient is to verbalize all the thoughts, emotions, and sensations that come to mind.

Furthermore, he is instructed to verbalize all these things freely, imposing no restrictions on himself. Once the patient is able to achieve this, he will experience the emergence of powerful emotions. This allows for a release of the unconscious feelings causing anxiety and possibly even mental and physical illness.

Additionally, these treatment sessions will continue until the effective expression helps the patient to release the repressed emotions and experience relief from anxiety. This can be particularly helpful to patients with back, neck, shoulder, and leg pain since these muscles are often adversely affected by nervous tension.

Covert Sensitization and Covert Behavior Rehearsal

First of all, covert sensitization is performed to change an unhealthy behavior that results in poor health. During this technique, the patient begins by visualizing herself participating in a behavior she wishes to change such as smoking or binge eating.

Next, the patient is instructed to abruptly follow this imagery with a mental picture of a devastating event that could result from the behavior. Of course, this causes the patient to associate the addictive behavior with a very unpleasant event, making it far less likely to occur in the future.

In addition, with covert behavior rehearsal, the patient is asked to repeatedly visualize the desired coping behavior. For example, athletes often use this approach by rehearsing the winning behavior in their minds before a big sporting event.

Moreover, while many visualization techniques are performed with the help of a therapist, there are also methods that can be performed by the patient alone.

Approximately 10 to 20 minutes in a relaxing atmosphere is all that is necessary to personalize imagery exercises to meet your individual needs.

Your Personal Visualization Session

Among several techniques that facilitate deep relaxation, visualization is one of the most effective. This is true because the brain operates on a highly visual level. For instance, if someone told you they bought a new car, you would most likely ask about the make and model. If you have seen a car like the one your friend purchased, your brain would "show you" a mental image of the car, which would bring about the next question: What color is it?

Therefore, since the human brain gravitates so strongly to images, it only makes sense that mental images can have a positive effect on mental and physical health. This is why visualization techniques are often implemented as a relaxation exercise geared toward eliciting the Relaxation Response.

While many visualization techniques are guided by a therapist, there are also exercises that can be performed by the patient on his own time. Opportunely, patients can use imagery to aid in their relaxation anywhere or anytime. A personal visualization session requires only 10 to 20 minutes in a comfortable environment. Once this is established, only a few simple steps are necessary.

Find a Relaxing Environment

To begin your imagery exercise, you must find a quiet place. If you are at home, go to a room where you are alone and not distracted by background noises like the television or your spouse talking on the telephone. Also, before starting your session, make sure you have 10 to 20 minutes to devote to relaxation. You want to be uninterrupted and able to reap all the benefits of deep relaxation. Next, make sure you are wearing comfortable clothing. This means clothing that is not too tight and also made of "breathable" fabrics such as cotton.

Choose the Image

When deciding upon an image, which basically the setting of your relaxation technique, it is important to choose an image that is both familiar and personal. For example, picturing yourself on a beach can be very calming and soothing. However, if you have never been to a beach, you might have to work harder to imagine yourself there.

Moreover, your image should be personal enough to initiate a pleasant emotional response. When your mind responds emotionally, it is easier to put yourself in the scene. Thus, you become part of it rather than just an observer. Most of all, your image does not have to include an exotic location. Instead, it should be a place that you enjoy and use to relax.

Develop the Image

Begin by using a familiar experience. For example, if you were on the swim team in high school, an image of your body gliding through the cool water can be used to provide the perfect visualization for relaxation. Of course, you would be better served if you imagined yourself swimming leisurely rather than sprinting.

This same principle holds true no matter what image you decide to use. In addition, it is also important to use all five senses. Continuing with the swimming example, the session would go something like this: Begin with the image, a lap pool. Most therapists encourage you to "sneak up" on the image.

So, imagine that you abruptly dive into the pool. As you resurface, *smell* the chlorine. *See* the small, white bubbles and bluish water moving smoothly around you as you look out through your goggles. All you can *hear* is the trickle as your *feel* your arms move in and out of the water, pushing it aside and propelling your body forward.

You also *hear* air going into your body as you turn your head sideways to take a breath. You *taste* a hint of cool water as some of it splashes into you open mouth. Then, as you exhale into the water, listen to the bubbles murmur past you. These are the only sounds you hear. All the other sounds are above the surface and separate from your watery world.

Develop A Technique to End Your Image

With any relaxation exercise, therapists recommend that you slowly allow normal thoughts to re-enter your mind. Thus, the transformation from deep relaxation back into everyday life should not be abrupt.

In the example that uses lap swimming as an image, you could imagine that you have decided to get out of the pool. Visualize yourself swimming over to a ladder located across the pool. As you swim to the ladder, you may begin to integrate your normal thought process.

Next, as you make your way over to the ladder and begin to step out of the water. Take the towel you have sitting near the pool and begin to dry off. And finally, make your way over to the locker room and get dressed. By the time you leave the locker room, you should be able to end the visualization session and go about the rest of your day.

Helpful Hints for Making Your Visualization Sessions Successful

Once you understand how to choose, develop, and end your image, you are well on your way to making successful visualization sessions part of your relaxation routine. Still, there are a couple of essential details to keep in mind.

For example, remember to use one image at a time. This allows for better concentration and deeper relaxation. Also, keep practicing your image. If you develop it enough, you will be able to use it as a cue for relaxation. For instance, if your image is the swimming pool, merely imagining it for a moment will calm you. Furthermore, it will become easier to relax each time you are "there."

Standard Imagery Exercises Pack A Big Punch

Though there are many different visualization techniques recommended to alleviate anxiety and ease back pain, some are more widely accepted than others. In fact, a few of these techniques have made their way into mainstream medicine.

They are used for pain management by patients with cancer and arthritis as well as women who plan to give birth without pain medication. Most importantly, they are beneficial for patients suffering from muscle pain, including back pain. Additionally, as with any visualization exercise, all you need is a tranquil environment and 10 to 20 minutes to yourself.

Passive Muscle Relaxation

This technique is beneficial for patients suffering from muscle pain, particularly back pain. Also, most people include passive muscle relaxation as part of their relaxation routine.

To begin this technique, imagine your muscles in a completely relaxed state. If it is easier, begin with your feet and progress upward until your face is also completely relaxed. No matter how you decide to visualize the relaxed muscles, remember that imaging loose muscles can be just as important as actually loosening them.

This is true because thinking about relaxing the muscles actually sends a signal to the brain. Once the muscles are relaxed, you may choose to implement one of the other relaxation techniques such as repeating a word, phrase, or physical motion. No matter what you decide, you should treat this imagery technique the same as any other.

Nevertheless, remain focused until you are prepared to slowly allow normal thoughts to re-enter your mind. Of course, it always helps to have an exit strategy. For this technique, you may find it helpful to count to three and then end with an affirmative statement such as, "I am relaxed and prepared to continue my day."

Additionally, you may have also heard of a technique called progressive muscle relaxation. This exercise isolates a particular muscle group and requires that the patient create tension in this specific group of muscles for approximately eight to ten seconds. The patient is then instructed to release the tension, allowing the muscles to completely relax.

The basic idea behind this technique is that the muscles relax after undergoing so much tension. Moreover, they are in a more relaxed state than before the exercise. Of course, this exercise is useful in isolating tense areas throughout the body; thus, it is effective in alleviating tension due to stress.

However, progressive muscle relaxation is not recommended for patients with strained muscles. In fact, for patients with back pain, it is contraindicated. Consequently, no matter what you friends or neighbors suggest, this exercise should be avoided if you have back pain.

The Beach Scene

This setting is often recommended by therapists who are coaching patients through imagery exercises. In many ways, this scene is ideal because it involves an image that is easy to develop. After all, it is a tranquil environment and finding images to satisfy all five senses is fairly simple.

Almost everyone can imagine the sensation of sand beneath his feet. What's more, even if you have never actually been to a beach, chances are that you have felt warm sunshine on your face and cool water on your hands. You might even be able to imagine salt in the air and the taste of fresh lemonade you might pack for a trip to the beach.

Moreover, many relaxation gadgets are equipped with noise which simulates the ocean waves. They may even have the distant calls of seagulls in the background. Most definitely, the beach scene is relaxing and inspiring. If you find that the beach is the right place for you to experience a deep sense of peace and elicit the mind-body connection, you should "go to the beach."

However, there are a lot of factors to bear in mind when it comes to achieving the deep tranquility it takes to promote mental and physical wellbeing. For instance, one of these is the emotional connection it takes for your mind to accomplish complete concentration. Thus, if you have more of an emotional connection with the pastures of the family farm, use that image instead.

Breathing Out Pain

This imagery exercise works well when used in conjunction with abdominal breathing, which utilizes all of the lungs and supplies muscles with nutrient-rich oxygen. If you were to use this technique to breathe out your back pain, the exercise would follow these basic steps: As you begin, take a few deep, calming breaths. You may find it helpful to count as you inhale and exhale, which will help to ensure that you exhale for twice as long as you inhale.

When you are ready, begin to add imagery to your breathing. You should start by visualizing fresh, cool oxygen going into your back muscles as you inhale. Furthermore, envision this oxygen delivering nutrients and comfort to the muscles. Then, begin to exhale and imagine the air leaving your back muscles, taking with it the pain and irritation.

Thus, all that remains is comfort, peace, and health. As you continue to breathe, imagine more and more comfort with each breath. After about 10 to 20 minutes, you should prepare to gradually end your breathing session. Many patients find that counting to three is a good way to transition from relaxation back to the normal thought process.

Understanding the Basic Theories of Hypnotism

Though experts cannot reach an agreement as to how hypnotism works, there are several theories that may explain its profound effectiveness. Nevertheless, evidence suggests that hypnotic therapy works by helping the patient focus his attention on achieving a desired outcome.

For example, when the goals are to find relief from back pain, hypnotism helps the patient concentrate on deep relaxation techniques such as mental imagery. Moreover, it also allows the patient to focus on suggestions made by the therapist. These suggestions can also be used to encourage certain behavior changes after the hypnotherapy session. Some examples of this include changes in eating patterns or ending harmful habits like cigarette smoking or alcohol abuse.

Furthermore, hypnosis may be used to promote positive behaviors, including athletes. While experts can only hypothesize on how exactly hypnosis works, there are several scientific theories. The theorists can be divided into two basic camps: state and non-state theories of hypnosis. Those who accept the non-state theories as the basis of hypnosis are convinced that focused attention and the amplified willingness to accept suggestions from a therapist. In contrast, those in the state theories camp believe that the foundation of hypnosis is an altered state of consciousness.

An altered state of consciousness can be defined as any condition that is substantially different from the normative waking beta state, which basically describes temporary changes to a person's mental state. These changes are induced; in some cases, they are induced by trauma, injury, or disease.

When participating in hypnosis, you are voluntarily entering a naturally occurring altered state of consciousness in order to find relaxation, encourage healing, or change a particular behavior. There are several distinct altered states of consciousness. These include dreams, lucid dreams, ecstasy, euphoria, and psychosis as well as premonitions, out-of-body experiences, and channeling. Still, whether you are inclined to side with the state theorists or the non-state researchers, it is beneficial to understand the various hypotheses and how they work.

Alpha and Theta State Theories

There are four unique brainwave patterns: beta, alpha, theta, and delta states. First of all, the alpha state is associated with relaxation and daydreaming. Many hypnotherapists suggest that this brainwave pattern is conducive to changing a patient's behaviors. This may include changes in eating habits, cessation of smoking or enhancing athletic performance.

Meanwhile, hypnotic therapists also believe that the theta state is permissive for therapeutic changes. This is due to the fact that sedatives, anesthetics and hypnosis disrupt a patient's neural synchrony; thus, neural synchrony is traditionally thought of as the basis for theta brainwaves.

Hypnotic techniques such as hypnoanalgesia and hypnoanesthia assist patients as they prepare for treatment, particularly minimally invasive treatments or surgical procedures. Furthermore, these methods occur more naturally in the theta and delta brainwave states.

Social Construction and Role-Playing Theory

The idea behind this theory is that hypnotism essentially does not exist. Proponents of the social construction and role-playing theory assert that participants go into the hypnotism session expecting to behave a certain way. After a meeting or two, the hypnotherapist is able to establish a rapport with the patient.

Social construction and role-playing theory advocates suggest that they become more open to the therapist's suggestions as a result. Meanwhile, there are research findings suggesting that a patient's expectations influence her hypnotism experience.

Still, this does not prove that hypnotism is little more that a game of role playing. This theory further proves the power of mental expectations when it comes to the effectiveness of hypnotism and how it facilitates mental and physical wellness.

Dissociation Theory

Supporters of these theories suggest that hypnotism is a form of dissociation from consciousness, which means that responses from the patient are automatic and reflexive.

Hypnosis as "Partial Sleep"

Some researchers have observed that some levels of hypnosis resemble the brain's waking state. Furthermore, many agree with this theory because the introduction to most hypnotism exercises involves closing the eyes. However, there are faults in the partial sleep theory because studies show EEG, blood pressure, and reflexes in most patients more closely resemble complete wakefulness.

Informational Theory

With this model, the hypnotherapist's goal is to use techniques that minimize interferences and make the patient more receptive to his suggestions. Thus, this theory likens the brain to a computer because such electric devices adjust feedback networks in order to raise the signal-to-noise ratio. This produces optimum functioning, which is also known as a "steady state."

Systems Theory

This theory serves as an extension of the original concept of hypnosis; thus, the systems theory asserts that hypnotism enhances or depresses nervous system activity. Hypnosis reorganizes the nervous system into interacting subsystems, changing not only the level of activity but also the cooperation among the subsystems.

Regardless of the theory to which you may subscribe, research suggests that hypnotic therapy is effective for many patients. It is effective for some more than others. This is most likely due to the fact that, contrary to popular stereotypes, hypnotism must be voluntary.

Furthermore, hypnotism is just one of the many exercises that demonstrate the power of the human mind. After all, just as the placebo effect illustrates, simply believing that a treatment will work produces results.

Hyper-Suggestibility Theorem

This increasingly popular theorem states that intense concentration amplifies the hypnotherapist's suggestions. Furthermore, this powerful focus on the therapist's words filters out anything that is irrelevant and allows the patient to concentrate on what is most important to her.

Your Guide to Understanding Hypnotherapy

Much like visualization techniques, hypnosis helps take the mind from its current surroundings into a deeply relaxed state. Though many people have misconceptions about hypnosis, it has become widely accepted by the medical community as a viable means of managing pain.

In fact, it is often used by patients with pain from surgery, chronic pain, nerve pain, and even childbirth. Nevertheless, it has many medical uses not related to pain. For instance, hypnosis can also be used to control addictive behaviors such as overeating, smoking, alcohol addiction, and drug addiction. Additionally, many patients rely on hypnosis to control anxiety, which often translates to physical pain, especially if it is repressed.

What You Can Expect from A Typical Session

A hypnotic session begins when the hypnotherapist guides the patient into an altered state of consciousness. At this point, the patient is focused and completely relaxed. Then, the practitioner will describe relaxing images and make suggestions on how to realize certain goals.

These may include things like alleviating pain or anxiety as well as refraining from unhealthy habits like smoking or overeating. Moreover, the hypnotherapist may use a technique during which she encourages the patient to focus on certain stimuli. For example, hypnotherapists often recommend certain mental images for the patient to visualize.

This method is particularly effective when the patient wishes to accomplish a specific goal. For instance, hypnosis combined with mental imagery is exceptionally beneficial for athletes interested in improving performance.

And finally, once a patient has experience guided hypnosis, she may have the opportunity to learn self-hypnosis. This technique can be taught by a professional hypnotist or self-taught with the appropriate literature or the help of a qualified professional. Furthermore, a self-hypnosis session is not altogether different from guided hypnosis.

Here is how it works: In order to prepare for self-hypnosis, it is best to choose which tools will be used during the session. For example, patients may use for themselves relaxing visualization techniques, word repetition, or affirmations such as "I am strong. I can handle the challenges of this ordeal."

Furthermore, self-hypnosis begins with a tranquil, comfortable environment free of distractions. Therefore, it is also essential to plan for 15 to 30 uninterrupted minutes of hypnosis. The next step is to become deeply relaxed; thus, some people count backward from a very high number (perhaps from 100) or imagine that they are gradually sinking downward.

Once this very deep relaxation is achieved, the patient may use one or more of the relaxation tools previously selected. And lastly, the conclusion of this session is similar to its beginning. Patients simply imagine that they are rising or waking. Next, they will make a suggestion like, "I will open my eyes, invigorated and alert." Of course, the patient will then open her eyes and resume all normal activity.

Hypnotism Is Still a Mystery

Even though this technique is accepted by the very skeptical medical community, experts have yet to reach an agreement on how it works. However, many practitioners do agree on several hypotheses. Practitioners know that hypnosis helps the patient experience deep relaxation and concentration.

Many suggest that hypnosis distracts the brain by redirecting its attention on something other than the pain, which would explain why mental imagery is so useful during hypnosis. Meanwhile, some believe that the patient is so deeply relaxed that the pain itself actually decreases.

Nevertheless, this makes sense when explaining pain relief experienced by patients with chronic muscle pain. Some theorize that hypnosis triggers the release of natural substances that affect the way the body senses pain. Still, others hypothesize that hypnosis works within the unconscious mind, which allows the patient to regulate heart rate, blood pressure, hunger, and other factors which the conscious mind does not control.

Why Hypnotic Therapy Is Misunderstood

When most people think of hypnotism, they recall comedy skits they have seen. Unfortunately, during these skits, the comedian most likely made the hypnotism into a charade. Though it may have been entertaining to watch a well-dressed, middle-aged man bark like a dog or jump around the stage like a chimpanzee, situations like these perpetuate the stereotypical misconceptions about hypnotism.

Contrary to popular belief, the hypnotist can not control your actions. You must be willing to be placed under hypnosis in the first place. Thus, the therapist simply makes suggestions, serving as a guide. Furthermore, you can not be placed in a hypnotic state against your will. In fact, even with voluntary participation, not all partakers are led into hypnosis.

Also, hypnotherapists also are confronted with the frightening myth that hypnosis can lead to amnesia. However, very few people encounter this problem. Even among those who do, these patients are always in a very deep hypnotic condition. Furthermore, they experience spontaneous amnesia, which usually lasts no longer than one day. Most of all, patients always have the ability to remember what took place during the hypnotherapy session.

Choosing a Qualified Hypnotherapist

Many healthcare practitioners in the field of medicine, dentistry, and psychology have hypnotherapy training in addition to their medical training. Meanwhile, even social workers have the ability to utilize this technique. On the other hand, certified hypnotherapy laypersons have acquired a specific amount of hours at a hypnotherapy school but have no additional medical expertise.

When looking for a hypnotherapist, take his training and experience into consideration just as you would when choosing a physician. For example, if you are looking into using a lay hypnotist, remember to inquire about the number of hours he trained, in addition to whether he is licensed by your state.

Nonetheless, it is very important to choose a highly qualified therapist because this form of therapy does carry some risk. For instance, if the hypnotherapist asks leading questions during the session, he can cause false memories to become implanted into your mind. Still, complications are very unlikely, especially when a reputable hypnotherapist is being used.

Biological Signals of Anxiety and Pain
Can Be Used to Your Advantage

There are many different causes of chronic back pain. In many instances, there is a specific problem that can be identified, such as muscle strain or nerve damage. In others, the body has simply become oversensitive to various stimuli. Psychophysiological assessments can usually identify causes of chronic back pain not diagnosable with other techniques.

For example, in low back pain, these assessments have the capability to detect abnormal patterns in which low back muscles interact with each other, as well as abnormal amounts of muscle tension. Furthermore, the combination of abnormal patterns and irregular amounts of muscle tension often trigger low back pain.

How Biofeedback Works

Biofeedback is a method that uses the mind to control a function that the body normally regulates automatically, such as skin temperature, muscle tension, heart rate or blood pressure.

When you are first learning biofeedback, you will have sensors attached to your body and to a monitoring device. These sensors are in place to provide instant feedback on the function being monitored. The biofeedback therapist will then teach you physical and mental exercises which can help you control the function. Furthermore, this is possible because the results are displayed on the monitor as you learn how to manage that particular function. And finally, the monitor beeps or flashes once you have accomplished the desired change in that body function, such as reducing muscle tension.

Most importantly, biofeedback is not hard to learn. In fact, training to use biofeedback requires only a few sessions in a biofeedback lab or other setting. Most people can achieve success with biofeedback with just a few sessions. Once they become well acquainted with this technique, they may use home biofeedback units.

With practice, many patients will be able to influence their muscle tension or blood flow without the help of the feedback monitor. In order to accomplish this, patients typically implement visualization techniques or a relaxation exercise such as deep breathing.

Patients learn how to identify the circumstances that trigger their symptoms and how to manage the stress of these events, which leaves the patient better equipped to deal with anxiety. Most are encouraged to change certain habits or to train in special techniques for gaining such self-control.

Studies have shown biofeedback to be very effective. In a study of patients with chronic back pain, they received 12 one-hour sessions of biofeedback. Then they were compared to a second group who received the same amount of treatment but were given false feedback. Instead of their own feedback, they were given the feedback taken from the muscles of patients.

The patients given accurate biofeedback reported at least a 40 percent reduction in pain intensity and half of them experienced a drop of 75 percent. Meanwhile, the other group reported no changes. Most importantly, the first group's improvements still held even after two-and-a-half years.

Biofeedback Technology

There are several different types of biofeedback machines that can provide information which can be helpful in identifying and reducing stress, anxiety, and tension that may be causing back pain. These include:

Electromyogram (EMG)   The electromyogram (EMG) measures muscle tension and is most often used to promote relaxation in muscles which have become tense in response to stress. First, two electrodes (or sensors) are placed on your skin over the muscle to be monitored. When the electrodes pick up on muscle tension, the machine gives you a signal, such as a colored light or sound.

During this process, you can see or hear continuous monitoring of your muscle activity and begin to focus on how the activity or tension feels. As you become more aware of this internal process, you will begin to recognize tension in your daily life. Then, you can make use of the techniques you learned in the biofeedback training to regulate the tension before it gets worse or causes other physical problems.

Temperature Biofeedback   This device monitors skin temperature. Furthermore, a sensor is usually attached to your foot or to the middle or small finger of your dominant hand. When you are tense or anxious, your skin temperature drops as blood is redirected inward to muscles and internal organs. Like monitoring muscle tension, measuring skin temperature is a useful tool in learning how to manage anxiety.

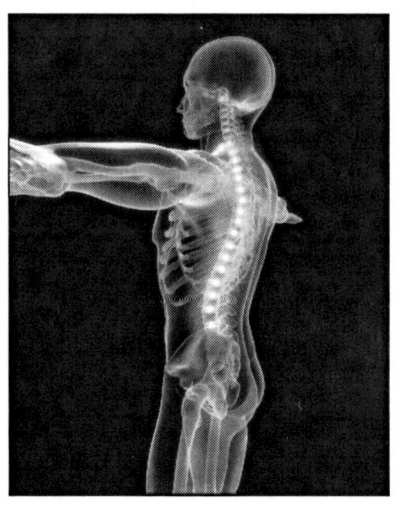

Galvanic Skin Response (GSR) or Electrodermal Response (EDR)   GSR measures electrical conductance in the skin, which is associated with the activity of the sweat glands. A very slight electrical current, unnoticeable to you, runs through your skin. Then the machine measures changes in the salt and water in your sweat glands. The more anxious you are, the more active your sweat glands are; thus, the electrical conductivity of your skin increases. Like many of these machines, GSR devices are designed to help determine and reduce anxiety.

Electroencephalogram (EEG)   This device monitors brainwave activity. As the brain emits electrical signals of various frequencies, the (EEG) breaks these frequencies into four classifications of brainwaves. First, beta waves are normally emitted when awake. Meanwhile, alpha waves are normally emitted during a state of calm relaxation and theta waves during light sleep.

Additionally, delta waves are given off during deep sleep. Since alpha waves are commonly observed during relaxation, the goal of reducing anxiety, stress, tension, and the back pain they can cause is achieved by learning to increase one's alpha wave activity. Still, alpha training is most effective when used in combination with other therapies.

All biofeedback devices are most effective when used in combination with relaxation techniques such as mental imagery and self-hypnosis. With biofeedback, you not only learn how to control your reactions to stress but also how you can explore the causes of stress, and your thoughts and behaviors that contribute to it. Of course, biofeedback is not magic. It cannot cure disease or, by itself, make a person healthy. Rather, it is one of many tools available to help you identify anxiety and learn how to manage it.

Biofeedback is a safe procedure and is most effective when taught by someone well-trained in biofeedback techniques. Of course, you should always tell your doctor before using biofeedback therapy by itself or in combination with other medical treatments. Moreover, biofeedback is not recommended for persons with severe psychosis, depression, or obsessional neurosis, nor for debilitated patients or those with psychopathic personalities. Additionally, it is contraindicated for use by diabetics and others with endocrine disorders because it can change the need for insulin and other medications.

Importance of Good *Posture*, Noun and Verb!

W hat's the first thing that comes to mind when you hear the word "posture"? Perhaps you recall your great-aunt telling you to "stand up straight," "keep your shoulders up," and "don't slouch." Or maybe you envision old movies in which ladies attending finishing school carefully practiced good posture by pacing the floor with a book balanced on their heads. You may possibly even think of your own posture and how you sit, stand, or walk.

Whatever imagery comes to mind, one thing that "posture" most likely does *not* conjure up is movement, and particularly energetic movement. Yet, as we are about to see, posture includes much more than uncomfortable, statuesque positions maintained for no purpose other than the ability to lay claim to "good posture"! How, then, can we categorize posture? Simply put, posture is either "static" or "dynamic." And understanding the difference between the two is the foundational starting point for recognizing how proper posture affects your body and can either cause or help alleviate back pain.

Before we can define static and dynamic posture, however, it is important first to define "posture" itself. Simply put, posture is the position or arrangement of the body and its limbs. The etymology of the word actually traces its line back through French and Italian to the Latin word *ponere*, meaning *to place*. Posture, then, is the placement of the body and its limbs at any given time.

Building on this foundation, we are now equipped to examine the two types of posture: static posture (SP) and dynamic posture (DP).

Static Posture

Static posture is defined as any posture or position held for a period of time. Particularly, then, static posture is the positioning of the body at rest, sitting, lying, or in an inactive standing position.

Static posture can be either natural or unnatural. For example, during sleep, the natural position of the body is by and large idle, with minimal movements. Likewise, when someone is resting or reclining in a chair or on a sofa, the body remains generally still, possibly with some occasional movement. When the body assumes this type of static posture, the muscles relax.

Not all static posture is natural, comfortable, or even healthy, however. When you position your body in a pose for a photo, you may be assuming a static posture that is temporarily uncomfortable but intended for a relatively brief period of time. For example, in the early days of photography, photographers would actually use braces to "prop" their human subjects up. These braces might support the back of a man's neck and include a rod extending down his back. Unquestionably, these were examples of unnatural static postures!

As in any unnatural static position, to keep a pose such as this, your muscles will tense, and blood flow may slow. Maintaining this type of unnatural static posture for an extended period of time will cause muscle fatigue resulting from the lack of blood flow, and the result of this can be discomfort at best and injury at worst.

Nevertheless, static posture is a natural part of body positioning. As we will see, however, it is only half the equation, and dynamic posture completes what is lacking by its static counterpart.

Dynamic Posture

If static posture is the positioning of the body at rest, then **dynamic posture** is essentially "everything else." More scientifically speaking, however, dynamic posture is the movement of any or all joints on a given axis of rotation. To put that into plain language, dynamic posture is the positioning of the body during movement.

The most obvious example of dynamic posture is sports. Imagine for a moment a runner racing around a track, a swimmer gliding through the water, or a goalie leaping in front of the goal. All of these athletes are exemplifying dynamic posture. Because every person is unique, the actual styles and manners of movement will vary from person to person – even among people doing the same thing. Two runners, for example, may run differently; two swimmers exemplify a different stroke style, and so on. Yet all of their movements fall into the category of dynamic posture.

It is not only athletic activities, however, that constitute dynamic posture. Movements as simple as walking, standing up or sitting down, climbing stairs, or getting in or out of a car or train are all examples of dynamic posture. And just as unnatural static posture can cause pain or even injury, unhealthy or careless dynamic posture can do the same.

For example, who hasn't heard of a friend "throwing his back out" while incorrectly lifting an object? Or of an athlete succumbing to injury as a result of an accident on the playing field? Or even of someone slipping down the stairs due to loss of balance? All of these injuries occurred while the body was practicing a "dynamic posture" activity.

Like static posture, dynamic posture is a natural part of body positioning and, just as its idle neighbor, it can be either healthy or unhealthy. The key is learning what constitutes healthy and unhealthy postures of both types and then committing to practice good postural habits. Your body will thank you!

Discover and Practice Your Ideal Static Posture

By now, we understand that static posture is any position of the body held for a period of time, such as standing, sitting, lying down, or reclining. While each of these has its principles and guidelines for what constitutes health and promotes overall bodily and skeletal comfort, for the purposes of this segment, we are going to focus on the basics of developing an ideal standing static posture.

Before we delve into the "how to," however, it's helpful first to understand the "why." Why is it important to develop healthful standing static posture? What benefits does it offer? Wouldn't it be just as good for each person just to adopt the standing posture that feels most "natural" to him or her?

First of all, healthful static posture *is* natural. What happens over time, however, is that the body often becomes lazy – both physically and mentally, and instead of positioning ourselves as nature intended, we adopt unhealthful posture. This can largely be due to the type of lifestyle that we live. Think about it. One hundred years ago, there were no computers to promote slouching, no escalators to allow us to "rest" while climbing stairs, no taxis to hail to avoid walking. The human body one century ago was in motion much more than the human body today. And while this may not automatically have translated into healthful posture, the lifestyle of enhanced movement made it harder to slip into poor posture habits.

So our goal is to re-adapt ourselves to a naturally healthful body posture. And, as we will see, the benefits are plentiful.

Healthful Static Posture Pluses

PLUS 1   An ideal standing static posture will keep bones and joints in healthful alignment. Not only will this ensure that there is no undue stress or pressure on our skeletal system and its connective joints, but it also allows the muscles to operate smoothly and normally without relying on excessive exertion to compensate for "out of whack" joints.

PLUS 2   An ideal standing static posture will prevent your muscles from becoming overly fatigued as a result of unnecessary exertion. Consider for a moment that if you are positioning your body in an unnatural standing position (i.e., shoulders slouched, hips jutting out, abdominal muscles lax), then other muscles in your body are working harder than necessary to balance out the "lazy" areas. And this can result in fatigue and undue stress on the muscles. Maintaining healthful standing static posture will help guard against this.

PLUS 3   An ideal standing static posture will protect your back and spine by preventing them from holding unusual or unnatural positions which can be detrimental to your health and your overall wellbeing. This protection also reduces the risk of back or muscle pain resulting from overuse, misuse, and excessive strain. Needless to say, no one wants back pain, so even if this were the only benefit offered by practicing healthful posture habits (which it is not), it would be well worth the effort!

Guidelines for Developing A Healthful Static Posture

We see the benefits of the ideal static posture, but how can we translate these benefits into reality in our everyday lives? By practicing the three Posture Principles. And, thankfully, they are quite easy to remember as each one is the same as the last!

Posture Principle #1 (and #2, and #3) – Alignment, Alignment, Alignment

If the key to selling real estate is location, location, location, then the key to developing the ideal static posture is alignment, alignment, alignment! Simply put, your skeletal system craves proper alignment in order to reduce skeletal strain, promote proper muscle functioning, and create a healthful internal environment for your body.

To check your alignment, concentrate on five focal points of the body: feet, knees, hips, shoulders, and ears.

- ❖ Your **feet** should be flat on the floor in a comfortable and neutral position. This provides a solid foundational point to support your entire skeletal system.

- ❖ Your **knees** should be straight, but not locked, and positioned directly above your feet.

- ❖ Your **hips** or pelvis should be in a neutral and level position, not tilted either forward or back and not jutting to one side. Slightly contract or tighten your abdominal muscles to support your lower back. This will feel a bit as if you are tucking in your stomach, but the ultimate purpose is proper body alignment.

- ❖ Your **shoulders** should be in line with your hips. Looking at yourself from the side, you should be able to draw a vertical line from your shoulders down to your hipbones. To do this, lift your chest and place your shoulders slightly back.

- ❖ Lastly, your **earlobes** should be aligned with the middle of your shoulders. Many people have a tendency to just their chins forward – in fact it is so common that in many cases we hardly notice it. By concentrating on lifting the head from behind and gently elongating the neck, we can keep the ears in line with the shoulders, and this not only contributes to healthful static posture but also actually increases the capacity for air flow into our lungs.

Now that you have the basics for developing an ideal standing static posture, there is only one thing left that you need. But don't worry – it's a tool that you already have right in your home. What is it? A mirror.

Just as with any skill or habit, developing an ideal standing static posture will take practice. But unlike other endeavors that require hours of rehearsal per day, at little as 3 or 4 minutes per day may be enough to effect a radical and healthful change in your body posture. Each day, set aside a few moments to evaluate your body posture. It may be in the morning as you prepare for your day or in the evening as you unwind. Whatever the time, take a few moments to stand in front of your mirror and assess your standing posture. Are your feet flat on the floor? Are you knees straight and relaxed? Is your pelvis evenly positioned? How about that tummy – is it tucked? Look at your shoulders, too. Are they aligned over your hips? And don't forget those earlobes! How are they positioned in relation to your shoulders?

If you invest just a little bit of time each day to ask yourselves these questions, before you know it, you will have developed the ideal standing static posture that is so important to overall skeletal health and wellbeing.

Healthy Sitting for a Healthy Back

Few activities in life are easier than sitting. In fact, sitting is so second nature that you may wonder why it merits the attention of an entire article. While it is true that sitting is indeed quite natural, the reality is that most of us are doing it wrong! And because in this highly computerized and technological age in which we live most of us are sitting more often and for longer periods of time than nature ever intended, we are reaping the negative results of our poor sitting posture.

The good news, though, is that by learning the do's and don'ts of healthy sitting, each person can assess his or her sitting habits, correct areas that need correcting, and develop a seated posture that is both comfortable and health-full!

A healthful sitting posture is one that allows the body to be properly aligned and places no undue stress on any of the muscles or joints of the body. Maintaining a healthy sitting posture offers both physical and non-physical benefits. *Physically,* you'll find that healthy sitting results in reduced instances of muscle and joint soreness, less skeletal stiffness, and fewer complaints of lower back pain. *Non-physically,* healthful sitting posture actually contributes to your mental ability to focus and be productive. If your body is comfortable and your muscles and joints are in alignment, you will be better able to focus on the tasks at hand without being distracted by aches, pains, or other physical discomforts. In short, a healthy sitting posture is definitely something to be pursued.

Eight Steps to Spectacular Sitting

What constitutes a healthy sitting posture? It is a combination of body alignment and body positioning. What follow below are eight simple steps that anyone can practice to develop a healthy sitting posture.

1. **One of the most common poor habits of sitting is the tendency to slouch.** The shoulders roll forward, the back curves, and the chest

collapses. To avoid this negative habit, sit down with the thought of sitting "up." Sit with your back straight and your shoulders slightly back. By focusing on what *to* do as opposed to what *not* to do, developing a healthful sitting posture can be a positive experience.

2. **Position your pelvis so that your buttocks touch the back of your chair.** This will provide much-needed support for your hips and lower back and will help ensure that you do not allow your hips to roll forward or backward, an almost sure sign of slouching.

3. **Curve that back!** *What? You* might be thinking. *I thought the back was supposed to remain straight!* Indeed it is, but by curving the back what is meant is simply maintaining the natural flow of the spine. A normally formed spine will have three curves, and each of these should be maintained while you are in the sitting position. To help keep your spine in its natural position, try placing a lumbar support or small rolled-up towel in the curve of your back. If your hips are positioned against the back of the chair, as mentioned above, this small towel will help you maintain proper spinal curvature.

4. **Keep your hips level and position your body evenly above your hips.** If you are leaning or "slouching" to one side or the other, your body weight will be unevenly distributed over your hips, making the muscles on one side of your body work harder than those on the other side, leading to discomfort, stiffness, or soreness. To avoid this, keep your body weight evenly distributed over your pelvis. If you are practicing the principle of sitting "up," even distribution of body weight will follow naturally.

5. **Place your feet flat on the floor.** For women especially, this may take the most effort. Many women have developed the habit, strengthened by years of practice, of crossing their legs. Although a widely accepted practice, leg-crossing is actually *not* healthy for your body! Not only can it restrict blood flow to the base leg, but it can also throw your pelvis out of alignment as it is nearly impossible to keep your body weight evenly distributed when one hip is higher than the other due to a crossed leg. So work on developing good sitting posture by keeping your feet flat on the floor.

6. **Adjust your chair height for proper line of vision.** If you work at a computer, as many people do, you should never have to look "up" to your computer screen as this will place stress on your neck. Similarly, your screen shouldn't be so low that you feel like you have to look excessively "down" to see it. Rather, your gaze should rest comfortably on the center of your computer screen.

7. **RELAX!** Few things are more detrimental to proper posture than tension. Stress from deadlines, work projects, and life in general can often cause us to tense our muscles without even realizing it. Sitting should not be a tense activity. So each time you sit down, take a moment to take a deep breath and relax your body. The release will do wonders for your muscles, joints, and skeletal system.

8. **Lastly, stand up.** While standing may sound as though it has little to do with a healthful sitting posture, in fact it has *everything* to do with it. Your body needs variety, and you should never sit in the same position for longer than half an hour. Make a decision that every 30 minutes you will pause in your work, stand up, and extend your back in a nice long stretch. Take a few steps – perhaps to a window or water cooler. If time permits, walk outside for 2 or 3 minutes. You will return to your work refreshed and rejuvenated.

By practicing these eight simple steps for assessing your sitting posture, you can develop healthful sitting habits that will promote comfort, productivity, and overall body wellbeing.

Simple Steps to Developing a Healthy Sitting Posture

When focusing on back health, posture is paramount to the discussion. Usually, the idea of posture brings to mind how one stands, walks, or carries herself. And, indeed, all of these do contribute to overall posture. But equally important to back health is sitting posture. In fact, with so many people working at desk jobs, often the amount of time one spends seated far outweighs time spent standing or walking. For this reason, developing a healthy sitting posture is vital to establishing a healthy-back lifestyle.

Sitting posture is simply defined as the way one holds his or her body while in a seated position. Yet many factors contribute to a healthy sitting posture, including body alignment, supportive chairs, and movement incorporation.

Body Alignment

Practicing proper body alignment is not difficult if you remember a few key points.

1. **Focus on keeping your shoulders back and your back straight.** This can be done using a simple head-chest-pelvis alignment test. Your head should be positioned above your chest, and both head and chest should be in line with your pelvis. If you find that your head is farther forward than your chest and pelvis, this is a telling sign that you may be slouching.

2. **Ensure that the very back of your pelvis touches the back of your chair.** If you find that there is space enough for your pelvis to roll back, in all likelihood you will soon find that it *is* rolling back and that you are falling into a slouched position.

3. **Remember that your back curves naturally, and all three of your normal back curves should be maintained.** In the absence of specifically designed lumbar support, a good way to check the natural curves of your back is to place a small, rolled-up towel in the lower curve of your back.

4. **Concentrate on keeping your body weight evenly distributed above both of your hips.** This is more easily done as you get into the habit of keeping the head-chest-pelvis alignment. Avoid leaning to one side or the other.

5. **Both of your feet should be positioned flatly on the floor.** Especially among women, there is the temptation to cross your legs. Although this is an extremely widespread practice, it does not ultimately contribute to a healthy sitting posture. Rather, your knees should be bent at right angles and should be positioned evenly or slightly higher than your hips. You may need to adjust your chair height to achieve this knee-hip alignment.

6. **If sitting in a swivel chair, turn your whole body instead of just turning at the waste.**

By doing this, you can maintain healthy alignment while still taking advantage of the benefits offered by pivoting chairs.

Supportive Chairs

Speaking of chairs, a properly designed chair can contribute greatly to a healthy sitting posture. There is no shortage of chairs claiming to provide excellent support and promote good posture, but what exactly should you look for when in the market for a supportive chair? Ideally, an effective and healthful chair will address several key areas of posture.

1. **Lower Back** As mentioned, proper posture includes maintaining the natural curve of your back, and a well-designed supportive chair will be constructed so it comfortably supports your lower back and causes it to arch slightly, keeping it in its natural "S" shape.

2. **Chair Height** While we often don't think of chair height as contributing to good or poor posture, in reality, it is a key factor. Your chair should be positioned at a level at which your eyesight gaze is directed at the center of your computer screen and your elbows, with hands rested on your desk as if typing, etc., are at a 90-degree angle. If you need to adjust your head to look "up" or "down" at your screen, or if your elbows are either overly bent or overly straight, then your posture is probably suffering, and you should adjust your chair to correct this.

3. **Calf Test** Perhaps you have a quality chair but are still feeling uncomfortable. If this is the case, it is possible that the chair is not properly adjusted. As mentioned above, your pelvis should be touching the back of your chair. From this position, perform the following simple test: Can you fit your fists easily between the front of your chair and the back of your calves? If the answer is no, then the chair depth is too great. This is often easily correctible, however, either through adjusting the back of the chair forward or by utilizing a lumbar support cushion or even a rolled-up towel to position your body farther forward in the chair.

Movement Incorporation

Even the best chair and ideal body alignment will not change the fact that we were not intended to sit indefinitely. And regardless of how healthy your sitting posture is, it is vital that you make a routine of getting up and moving around. A good rule of thumb is to take a "stretch break" once every 30 minutes. This may involve standing up and simply moving around for one minute or taking a brief walk to get some fresh air and a change of scenery. Movement not only increases blood flow in your body but also gives your joints a chance to stretch out, thereby providing increased comfort when you do return to a seated position.

As we as a population spend more and more time seated for work or entertainment, it is becoming increasingly important that we focus on the effects of our seated posture. And with the simple guidelines outlined above, you, too, can be on your way to adopting a healthy sitting posture.

Sleeping 101: Sleep Essentials for a Healthy Back

Chances are you never thought you'd be reading a "how-to" article on sleeping. After all, not even infants require instruction in the fine art of slumber! But even with hundreds and thousands of nights spent in practice, many men and women today are not reaping the benefits of healthy sleep. And much of this has to do with their sleeping posture.

More than just affecting the nighttime hours, the quality of your sleep affects every area of your life. Consider for a moment — have you ever tossed and turned for hours, unable to "get comfortable"? Have you ever awakened in the middle of the night for no apparent reason? Have you ever climbed out of bed in the morning only to wince because of a stiff neck or a sore back? After any one of these experiences, was your day as productive as it could have been? Or did you feel sluggish, fatigued, or generally out of sorts?

You see, healthy sleeping posture is vital both to ensuring proper rest and to preparing your body for the day's work. And when it comes to healthy sleeping posture guidelines, the two most important things to remember are position and surface.

Position

Many people debate the pros and cons of various sleeping positions. Is sleeping on your back best? Is it truly bad to sleep on your stomach? What about side sleeping? As in standing posture, the key factor when considering sleeping positions is alignment. You should sleep in such a way so that your skeletal system remains in a neutral and proper alignment without any undue stress falling on any one portion of your body.

The Back Sleeper

Many people opt for sleeping on their backs as the most comfortable position. Yet, if you're not careful, back sleeping can also be a breeding ground for injury and strain. This is because back sleeping creates the possibility for back over-extension. As in sitting, while sleeping you want to ensure that your back maintains its natural curve, and back sleeping is not always conducive to this.

This does not mean, however, that you must swear off sleeping on your back. With a few minor adjustments, you can comfortably and safely remain a back sleeper. The goal is simply to ensure that you provide your back with proper support. To do this, try placing a lumbar roll under your lower back or a pillow under your knees. Either of these will help position your body so that your back is well-supported and its healthy curves maintained.

The Stomach Sleeper

Of the three sleeping positions discussed here, the stomach position is the one that you should most avoid. And this is particularly true if you have an especially soft or sagging mattress. Due to lack of support for the core section of the body, stomach-sleepers place excessive stress on their lower backs. Over time, this can cause back strain and even neck pain as the effects of lack of back support extend beyond the immediate lower-back area. If at all possible, avoid sleeping on your stomach.

The Fetal Position Sleeper

It is for good reason that the majority of people favor the fetal position as their sleeping position of choice. Not only is this position the most natural but of all the sleeping positions, it also offers the greatest benefits for postural health. However, there are a few things to remember when sleeping in the fetal position.

First, remember, that sleeping in the fetal position is *not* the same as merely sleeping on your side, and, in fact, individuals who sleep on their sides with their legs extended straight causes their pelvis to be positioned out of alignment and places stress on their lower back. Rather, your knees should be bent (although not too tightly crunched). In addition, to provide the greatest support for your hips and backs, try placing a pillow between your knees. This will keep your back and spine in a neutral position and help prevent misalignment, injury, and pain.

Surface

Equally important to body positioning is the surface on which you sleep. Far too many people pay far too little attention to this, and the result is poor sleep, aches and pains, and the potential for long-term injury.

Beds

To avoid these pitfalls, it is imperative that you **invest** in a good bed and mattress. Consider the bed frame *construction*. Is it stable? Is it well-made? Remember, price may not always be an indication of quality, so avoid **purchasing** a more expensive bed frame simply because you are equating price with quality. The more expensive one may end up being the best choice, but if it is not, don't be afraid to shop around.

Ensure that you purchase a mattress and box spring set that provides firm support and will not sag. One tip to prevent sagging is to place a board underneath your mattress between the mattress and the box spring. Saggy mattresses are a sure way to promote back stress, so avoid them at all cost!

While soft mattresses may seem more comfortable at first, they do not provide the best support for your back. If selecting a too-firm mattress is too uncomfortable for you, then go a bit softer, but be sure your mattress maintains enough firmness to provide adequate support.

Couches

This article would be incomplete without a word on couch sleeping. Naturally, a couch is not the ideal place to sleep. Couches are not designed or manufactured with sleep-style spinal and lumbar support in mind. Nevertheless, all of us will occasionally take an afternoon nap on our living room couch. And when we do, we can still do something good for our posture by taking time to select a supportive pillow. The pillow should support your neck properly and, as much as is possible, keep your neck in line with your spine. Although a couch does not provide the supportive benefits of a well-made bed, by maintaining spine-neck alignment you can still give your body a healthy-lift even when napping on the living room sofa!

Remember, you may spend as much as one-third of your life sleeping! Do something good for yourself by making the decision to practice healthy sleeping habits.

Dynamic Posture: Guidelines for Assessment

Dynamic posture, or the positioning and flow of our body during movement, plays a vital role in our skeletal health and comfort. While a poor dynamic posture can lead to strain, sprain, and even injury, a proper dynamic posture can promote strength, flexibility, airflow, and general wellbeing.

But what actually constitutes a "proper" dynamic posture? After all, the number of movements a person completes in a single day is probably too high to be counted.

Indeed, while dynamic posture varies from activity to activity and even from person to person, for our purposes we will examine proper posture for walking. From head to toe, we will highlight four areas of assessment for determining if you are practicing a healthy dynamic posture.

Head Position

Proper head positioning while walking is essential to maintaining a healthy dynamic posture. Your head should be forward-looking, with your gaze resting approximately 20 feet in front of you. If you are constantly looking down at your feet, you cause extra strain to be placed on your neck. In addition, the rest of your body will more than likely follow your eyes' gaze; a downward gaze will cause your shoulders to slouch, having a detrimental effect on your entire body positioning. A raised head and forward-looking gaze, however, will encourage a natural effect of lifted chest, squared shoulders, and healthy body alignment. If you're unsure of this, try it. Try to slouch your shoulders while keeping your head and eyes raised; it's difficult to do, right? The first step toward assessing your dynamic posture, then, is considering the position of your head.

Stomach Stability

Next time you're walking down the street and you pass a storefront window, look at yourself and watch your body alignment. Are you "sitting" in your pelvis with your stomach jutting out? If so, you are placing undue stress on your lower back. Whereas some people may think that we tuck our tummies in only for vain purposes, the truth is that keeping our abdominal muscles slightly contracted provides support for our lower backs. So take an honest look at yourself in that display window and if your stomach is lax, tighten it up.

Examine Your Step

Walking should be a fluid motion, with minimal jarring and pounding on any of your joints — ankles, knees, hips, etc. We've all noticed some people, however, whose walk precedes them via sound waves! These people may be either lightweight or heavy, as weight is not the determining factor here. The one thing they have in common is the force with which their feet strike the floor, each step a loud and jarring pounding motion that threatens to leave a dent at the point of impact! While some people may recognize their heel-pounding action, others may be completely unaware of it. And this goes for anyone reading this article, too! Are you a heel pounder?

If you want to ensure that you are not, return to that shop-front display window and observe yourself walking. Does your head bob up and down with each step?

Does each stride seem to involve equal vertical movement as horizontal, forward movement? Can you "feel" each heel strike up through your legs? If so, then you may be an unknowing offender in the heel-pounding category.

To correct this malady, simply remember the heel-roll-toe principle of walking. Your heel-strike is only the first component of a smooth walking stride. Rather than stop at the initial strike, your foot should roll gently forward through the insole and to the ball, ending with a push-off from your toes. Now, try that and watch yourself again in the window. Do you see a difference? Chances are that you do.

Foot Flare

An often unmentioned factor of dynamic posture assessment is the presence of "foot flare." Simply defined, foot flare is the degree to which someone's toes point outward when he or she walks. Healthy foot positioning means that both feet are facing forward with your toes pointing forward, and only a slight toe-out position if any. The presence of significant foot flare, however, may be an indication of a problem in the lower back or hip areas.

To assess if foot flare is present in your walking gait, simply walk normally and observe your feet. Since you're now aware of foot flare, it may be easy to force your feet to point forward, but it's important that you avoid doing this as you assess your true dynamic posture. If after an honest assessment you notice foot flare, a chiropractor can provide further evaluation of your hips and spine in relation to the foot flare.

While everyone's dynamic posture is unique, and while such posture varies greatly with different movements, by honestly evaluating your own dynamic walking posture, you will be able to identify any areas needing improvement and you will be able to make the needed adjustments to provide the greatest level of support for your muscular and skeletal system.

Healthy Walking:
The Seven Habits of Highly Effective Walkers

It's one of the most natural things we do. From sunup to sundown, chances are none of us even thinks twice about it. And yet this simple action we call walking exerts tremendous pressure on our bodies.

Experts estimate that the average person takes approximately 5,000 steps per day — and this figure is calculated based on a fairly *sedentary* lifestyle. This means that just by going about your daily business – walking around your house, to and from your car, to and from the bus or train stop, around the office, etc. — you may be taking as many as 35,000 steps per week. And pound for pound, each step places a pressure on our body at the rate of three times our body weight! With these statistics, it is no wonder so many people experience feet, back, and overall skeletal discomfort after periods of walking.

But it doesn't have to be so. Our bodies, after all, were created for movement and were intended to walk. The problem, then, lies not in the activity of walking itself, but in *how* we are walking. In order to maximize body efficiency while minimizing any pain or discomfort associated with this all-natural movement, it's important to understand the habits that contribute to healthy walking.

These can easily be remembered as the **Seven Habits of Highly Effective Walkers**.

Shrug Your Shoulders

Because your entire body is interconnected, walking involves much more than just your feet! The first habit that healthy walkers embrace, then, is maintaining an uplifted posture. The term "uplifted" is used here instead of "straight" as straight often implies "stiff." Your walking posture should not be stiff, but your shoulders should be slightly back. To avoid stiffening, shrug your shoulders once and then let them relax. Perfect!

Eyes Straight Ahead

It may seem unusual to relate your eyes to healthy walking posture, but the level of your gaze plays an important role in the positioning of your head. Because of this, you should keep your eyes looking forward with your gaze aimed approximately 20 feet in front of you. If your eyes are constantly directed down toward the ground, your head will soon follow, creating undue stress on your neck and, by extension, your back.

Tuck In That Tummy

While this may sound rather vain at first, in reality it has nothing to do with vanity and everything to do with your health. By slightly tightening your abdominal muscles while walking, you are actually supporting your lower back. When our abdominal muscles are too relaxed as we walk, the relaxation can actually cause us to begin to arch our backs as our stomachs come forward. Tighten up your abdominal muscle wall, even just a bit, and you will do wonders toward lessening the strain on your lower back.

The Perfectly Placed Pelvis

We've talked about your head, shoulders, and tummy, but several of the main skeletal "hinges" your body uses when walking are actually in your pelvis. It's important that when you walk, your pelvis remain level. While this may sound easy and natural enough at first, in reality, many people do not keep a level pelvis when they walk. Think for just a moment. Have you ever seen someone walking who seems to be "leading with his or her hips"? Their posture is such that they are "sitting in their hips." And, if you'll continue to watch them, as they walk you will notice excessive movement in their pelvis.

Remember when we said that all of the body is interconnected? This holds true with the pelvis, too. And pelvic instability often means poor posture in other areas. (If someone is "leading with the hips," it's likely that his or her shoulders are also not lifted.) Concentrate on keeping a level pelvis, and you'll be practicing one of the seven habits of highly effective walkers!

Be a Smooth Operator

This all-important habit means that walking should be a smooth activity. Remember, walking is natural! So there should be no sudden jerks in your stride. This does not mean that everyone's stride will be the same or even similar. Some walkers may have a long stride that seems to carry them the length of a room in three steps, while others may need to take five steps just to keep up to another's one. There is no "right" walking style. As long as your stride is smooth and comfortable, you're on the right track.

Walk on Clouds

Perhaps this is a bit of an exaggeration, but by walking on clouds, the idea is that there should be no jarring or pounding with each step you take. To practice this habit, try to think of walking as movement directed *forward* rather than movement directed *up and down*. Up-and-down walkers tend to pound the floor with each step, and their movement is not fluid. Forward walkers, however, seem almost to sail over the floor. How do they do this? It's simple, really, if you remember the little phrase of "heel-roll-toe."

Each step begins with your heel coming into contact with the ground first. Then, your foot should roll through the length of your insole and through to the toe. Push off the ground with your toe and repeat the process with the other foot. The whole movement should be gentle and light. Think of your foot as sinking into a soft cloud rather than striking a hard floor. By concentrating on this simple heel-roll-toe method, you'll minimize harmful jarring and create a walking style that is healthy both for your feet and for your entire body. With just a bit of practice, smooth walking will soon become second nature.

Bid Tension "Ta-Ta"

Finally, remember that walking is one of the most natural movements that our bodies do. And while all of the tips provided here are important to developing healthy walking habits, make sure that they don't become a walking "to-do" list that transforms the activity from relaxing recreation to tension-filled practice sessions. Rather, keep all of the tips in mind, but before you take a step, take a deep breath and exhale. Think about releasing the tension of the day from your body. You will find that with a relaxed body, it is much easier to remember the habits of keeping a level pelvis, walking smoothly, and holding your head up.

And by practicing these Seven Habits of Highly Effective Walkers, you will be treating your body to one of the most natural and healthy activities in the world.

Happy Walking!

Not All Shoes are Created Equal!
How to Buy The Right Shoes for Healthy Posture

At the beginning of time, men and women lived off the earth, maintained healthy organic diets, and walked barefoot through lush grass and vegetation. Ah, paradise! At least in some ways. Granted, today we enjoy additional simple pleasures in life such as, oh, the wheel, for example, but we no longer run barefoot through the meadows. Instead, we pound our bodies daily by striding on concrete, running on asphalt, racing up and down stairways, and simply walking around our homes. And all of these things can potentially affect our body's health and comfort.

It's been estimated that the average person will walk approximately 115,000 miles in his lifetime. That's the equivalent of walking around the Earth's equator more than four times! And every step we take places a pressure on our feet of up to three times our body weight. This means the feet of a 150-pound person absorb as much as 450 pounds of pressure in every step of the 115,000 miles!

With such a pound-for-pound impact, it's understandable why our bodies — and especially our feet and backs — begin to "feel it" when we're on our feet for extended periods of time.

How Our Feet Work

Next time you take a step, pause for a minute to consider the anatomy of the movement. Your heel will strike the ground first, followed by a rolling motion through which the rest of the foot hits the ground from heel to forefoot. If shoes do not properly support this movement, back pain can result. This is especially true with high-heels. Heels can pull your entire body weight forward, thus placing additional stress on the arches of your back.

In short, if shoes aren't providing the proper support, it's no wonder that aches and pains appear in the skeletal system.

But there is hope. Proper shoes are available that provide vital support and aid in shock absorption, thus lessening the pressure on our bodies. And with just a bit of time and effort, you can find the pair of shoes suited to your feet and body type. So what should you look for when buying shoes? Read on!

The Shoe Factors: Heel, Flexibility, Insole, and Toe

Heel Since the heel is the first part of your foot to strike the floor, let's start there. You should purchase shoes only after paying close attention to the fit in the heel. Experts recommend that the heel fit be snug and create a solid support. If there is too much space in the heel, the initial impact of your foot hitting the ground (or pavement, floor, concrete, etc.) will not be well supported. The fit should be snug yet comfortable in order to provide maximum support and guidance for feet as you walk.

Flexibility We've all endured a pair of shoes that felt like more like concrete blocks than footwear! And naturally, stiff, inflexible shoes can wreak havoc on your feet and your posture as they don't allow for any "give." The human foot is not static but dynamic, and a good shoe will reflect this. If a shoe does not bend at all when you walk (or worse yet, if you can't bend it by hand!), then put it back on the display shelf and move on. For further proof of the importance of flexibility, consider it in relation to the next shoe factor: insole.

Insole Considering the way a shoe fits in the arch of your foot is vital to purchasing good shoes. But how do you do this? First, it is important to determine the type of arch you have — whether low or flat, medium, or high. A good way to do this is to dip your bare foot in water and then step on a towel. What kind of imprint did your foot leave? Did the mid-section of your foot leave a wide mark? Perhaps even close to the width of your heel? If so, you have a **low arch**. If the arch imprint is about half the width of the ball of your foot, then you have a **medium** arch, and if you can only see a thin line where your arch hit the towel, your arch type is **high**.

The insole of your shoe should provide adequate support for your arch type. If you have a high arch, for example, you'll want to avoid shoes with flat insoles, as these will not properly support your feet when you walk. Likewise, if your feet are flat, a high-arched shoe will place undue pressure on your foot, potentially causing discomfort and poor walking mechanics.

Toe   We've made it from the heel through the insole and have arrived at the toe. The most obvious guideline here is to ensure that you don't purchase shoes that are too small length-wise. Beyond this, however, it's also important that your shoes not be too small width-wise or even height-wise. Your toes should never be constricted to the point of pain. This is particularly true when purchasing athletic shoes, and when buying shoes for sport or exercise, always make sure that your toes have a bit of "wiggle room."

There are countless shoes out there in the world – and with many stores offering sales, discounts, and buy-one-get-one-free deals, it's all too easy to place pocketbook above posture. But your body deserves better! Make the decision to buy only those shoes that provide proper support. Believe me, your feet and back will thank you!

Keep Your Back Intact Part I: The Six "Don'ts" of Lifting and Bending

Each of us has at some point or another been faced with the task of lifting a heavy object. Perhaps you were moving a box of books or souvenirs into storage, rearranging furniture, or moving materials as a part of your job. Whatever the scenario, if you are not careful, lifting heavy objects can quickly lead to back injury ranging from minor to severe.

To reduce chances of injury and keep your back intact, it's vital to understand both the DOs and the DON'Ts of lifting heavy objects. This piece will focus on the six things to avoid at all cost when lifting and bending. Remember, it only takes one slip-up to cause an injury that can potentially last a lifetime. To avoid such an injury, make sure you also *always* avoid the following missteps:

1.   **DON'T keep your feet close together.**   One of the most important elements of healthy lifting and bending is balance. If your feet are touching or positioned closely together, you have ceded this vital element. The principle is a simple one. Think for a moment of trying to position a wooden pole upright without rooting it in anything. More likely than not, the pole may remain upright for a second or two and then slowly begin to lean to one side. It quickly gains momentum and slices through the air to land with a thud on the ground. It had no solid foundation. Now consider balancing the same

pole if it is attached to a wide base on the bottom. Suddenly, what was once a daunting task becomes simple. The base provides stability, and the pole stays erect. Positioning your feet too close together makes you like that pole in the first example – without a base and easily swayed.

2. **DON'T bend at the waist.** We've all been given this advice. But have you ever stopped to think of *why* you shouldn't bend at the waist when lifting a heavy object? Your waist is not your strongest bodily lever. In fact, because many people have not developed a strong core section, meaning strong lower back and abdominal muscles, your midsection can often have hidden weaknesses. Bending at the waist places the bulk of the weight of the load on your lower back, and trying to lift an object while doing this can easily cause back strain or even more serious injury.

3. **DON'T lift objects that are too heavy for you.** Regardless of how much you may want to impress your peers, lifting objects that are too heavy is simply too dangerous to be worth it! Be honest with yourself concerning your strength level.

4. **DON'T lift objects that are far away from your body.** Like bending at the waist *reaching* and *lifting* together form a dangerous duo. It's impossible to maintain a safe and healthy body position if you are extending your arms far in front of you to lift an object. It places far too much strain on the lower back and poses the added danger of causing you to lose your balance. Remember, if it's too far in front of you, it's too dangerous to lift.

5. **DON'T lift and carry an imbalanced load.** Even if an object is not too heavy for you to lift, pay careful attention to how the weight of the object is distributed. If it is unevenly balanced, your muscles will have to overcompensate in order to maintain your balance *while* still exerting effort to keep the object lifted and carrying it from point A to point B. With a simple misstep, an unevenly distributed load can lead to loss of balance, tripping, falling, and serious injury.

6, **DON'T lift and bend repetitively.** Although the body is perfectly engineered for movement, it also requires rest. And repetitive lifting and bending without providing adequate time for muscles to rest and recover can open the door to muscle pain, strain, and even serious injury. Despite the fact that rest is essential, the reality is, however, that some people are required to bend and lift constantly simply because of the nature of their jobs. Perhaps they work in building and construction, or at a dockyard, or in landscaping. For these workers, bending and lifting are necessary parts of their day. This does not mean, however, that they should not give their bodies rest. Taking mini-breaks throughout the day and stretching muscles can provide much-needed rest and relief. In addition, even teaming up with fellow-workers to lift particularly heavy loads together can lessen the stress and strain for those whose livelihood requires regular lifting and bending.

By avoiding these six *Don'ts* of bending and lifting, you will avoid painful and dangerous injuries. So "don't" forget to avoid the "don'ts", and you won't be faced with an unwanted accident or injury!

Keeping Your Back Intact Part II: The Seven "Do's" of Lifting and Bending

"Lift with your legs!" We've all heard that admonishment before, usually just *after* we've improperly bent at the waist and hoisted up a heavy box. By then, of course, it was too late. If only we'd remember the legs *before!*

Whether the object to be moved is a box, a table, or even your active little toddler, maintaining proper posture and movement while lifting and bending is paramount to protecting your back and reducing the chance of injury. Just as it's vital to avoid the six "don'ts" of lifting and bending, it's equally important to practice the six "do's" of healthy lifting and bending. And the good news is that they are not all difficult to master.

1. **DO place your feet at the proper width apart.**   Your feet are the starting point for safe lifting posture. They do, after all, form the foundation that sets the stage for the placement of your entire body! To ensure maximum safety and stability while lifting, your feet should be positioned in a semi-side stance, about shoulder-width apart. Make sure that your feet are firmly planted, and never, NEVER attempt to lift or carry heavy objects while wearing high-heels.

2. **DO use your legs when lifting.**   Perhaps the worst mistake people make when lifting heavy objects is keeping their knees straight while bending at

the waist. This can be a sure sign of an impending injury. Instead, when lifting an object from the floor or a surface lower than your waist, bend at the knees and at the hip joints (not waist) in order to position yourself to lift the object. Once you have a firm grasp on the object, push up *through your heels* extending your knees and hips until you are back in a standing position. Once standing, it's important not to lock your knees as this will compromise your balance. And remember, when putting the object down, these same principles hold true – just in reverse order!

3. **DO keep the weight of the object close to you as you lift.**   Just as it's dangerous to try to lift an object that is far away from you, so, too, it is dangerous to try to extend an object away from you after you have lifted it. Pushing a heavy load away from you may easily cause you to lose your balance, drop the load, or, worse yet, fall. By keeping the object close to your body, you are keeping it close to your center of gravity, and it will be much easer to transport it. Not only this, but your muscles and joints have to work harder the farther away an object is placed from your body. Imagine your body as a fulcrum and your arms as levers. The farther away a weight is from the fulcrum, the greater the stress and strain on the levers. So give your body a break and keep your load close to you!

4. **DO carry a balanced load.**   Few things can throw your body off balance more quickly than a load that is unbalanced or constantly shifting. To protect your muscles and joints and maintain your balance, ensure *before* you lift the object that the contents are balanced and the weight is evenly distributed. If the contents are such that they might shift during movement, take an extra few minutes to stabilize them by adding package fillers or even by breaking down the load into two separate, smaller loads. The few minutes spent on ensuring balance may spare you weeks or longer of injury recovery.

5. **DO avoid lifting objects above waist-level.**   Whenever you lift an object above waist level, you are automatically placing increased stress on the lower back. Particularly if someone has a weaker lower back or a history of back pain or injury, such lifting can be extremely dangerous. When you lift an object, then, make sure that you never lift it higher than waist level. If you find that you must raise an object higher, then *get help!* Either utilize a mechanical device or, if that is not an option, call for reinforcements! Regardless of how

inconvenient it may seem to solicit the help of others, it's far more inconvenient, and potentially very long-term, to have to deal with a back injury.

6. **DO push rather than pull.**   If you find that you have to move an object – either on the floor or on a raise surface — always *push* the object rather than *pull* it. When you pull, not only are placing undue strain on your muscles but you are also putting yourself in a position in which it is easy to lose your balance. Pushing, however, gives you the benefit of being able to put your whole body weight behind the effort and makes it much easier for you to protect your back. Moreover, if you lose your balance, it's unlikely that you will go crashing to the floor.

7. **DO pay attention to maximum lifting guidelines.**   Even if you believe you can lift more than the guidelines allow, *don't do it!* Remember, these safety guidelines are there for a reason, and that reason is to protect you and your back and muscles from unnecessary injury.

At one point or another, nearly every person will be faced with the task of lifting a heavy object. While for some it may be a constant requirement of a job, for others, it may be a one-time task. Whatever the situation, by following the seven guidelines for healthy bending and lifting, you can practicing safe lifting methods, complete your task, and keep your back intact!

Building a Better Back:
Exercises to Promote Back Health

Turn on any television set at any given time, and you're likely to see several info-mercials advertising the latest in exercise and strength training equipment. While some of the items have more merit than others, all of the advertisements tout the importance of physical exercise to good health. And they are right, for regular exercise is a necessary component of any healthy lifestyle.

When many people think of exercise, however, they think of cardiovascular exercise such as jogging, biking, or swimming, or of weight exercises to strengthen those biceps, triceps, and legs. Unfortunately, too many people omit from their exercise regimen one of the most important parts of the body: the core.

Your core muscles include you abdominals and lower back, and these muscles are involved in virtually every movement your body makes. From standing up and sitting down to walking down the street, to lifting objects, to turning from side to side, all of these movements engage the core muscles. It's obvious to see, then, why it is important to develop strong and healthy core muscles and also why weak core muscles can contribute to pain and discomfort. This is particularly true when it comes to back pain.

Back pain — and especially lower back pain — is often a result of a weak lower back. While we spend so much time doing those arm curls, we often neglect to strengthen our lower backs. Because of this, they are more susceptible to injury and strain. Yet, even though so many of us neglect our backs, developing a strong core section does not have to be difficult.

There are several simple exercises for strengthening your back that can be performed right in the comfort of your own home. And if you currently have a healthy back, congratulations, but don't use that as an excuse *not* to exercise your back. Even healthy men and women should make a determined decision to increase back strength because in doing so they can help prevent future back injuries and back pain.

If you are currently suffering from back pain or a back injury, back exercises can often help speed recovery and prevent future injury. Always consult with your medical professional first, however, before beginning any back exercise program.

The following are five easy-to-learn, beginning lower-back exercises that anyone can do. These exercises require minimal equipment – in fact, only a towel or a mat to lie on will be sufficient. As with any exercise, the movements should not cause pain, and if you experience pain, stop immediately and consult a healthcare professional.

Knees-to-back Lower Back Exercise and Stretch

Lie on your back on a firm surface. Place your towel or mat on the surface for added support and comfort. Your legs should be extended flat on the floor. Slowly bring one knee to your chest. Clasp your hands behind your thigh and gently pull the knee in to your chest. Hold this position for 30 seconds. Remember to continue to breathe. Slowly release your leg and return it to the starting position. Repeat with opposite leg. To vary this exercise for a maximum lower back stretch, slowly bring BOTH legs together to your chest and hold for 30 seconds. You should feel a nice stretch in your lower back.

Cat and Camel

Kneel on the floor for the starting position. You should be on all fours. Keep your head in line with your back so your gaze should be directed toward the floor. Slowly round your back at the waist while contracting, or tightening, your abdominal muscles to provide back support. Your head will fall slightly forward as you do this movement. From this position, slowly lower your back and arch it so that it dips in the center toward the floor. Your head will come up a bit (although not too much as this will strain your neck). This arched position should be comfortable and not feel "forced." Again, remember to breathe during the motion.

Back Extension

Lie on your stomach on your mat or towel. If you are a beginner, select option A below. If you are more advanced, select option B.

    A.   Place both hands, palms down, under your shoulders. Slowly push your upper torso up while keeping your pelvis on the floor. Your back will be arched (again, be sure you don't feel pain). Hold this position for 10 to 12 seconds and then return your torso to the floor.

B. Place both arms straight by your sides. Without the aid of your hands or arms, slowly lift your head and shoulders off the mat. You do not need to lift them very high, just to a point that is comfortable for you. Slowly return to the starting position.

Hip Extension

Lie on your stomach on the mat or towel. Bend one leg so that your knee is at a 90-degree angle and your foot faces the ceiling. Gently lift that leg toward the ceiling, pressing up through the heel. The movement will be very small — only a few inches — and concentrated. Be sure to keep your hips in contact with the floor throughout the movement. Slowly lower the leg to the starting position. Repeat with opposite leg.

Abdominal Curl

The abdominal muscles are the opposing muscle group to the lower back. Because of this, it is important that any exercise program for the back also involve the abdominals so a balanced level of strength is achieved.

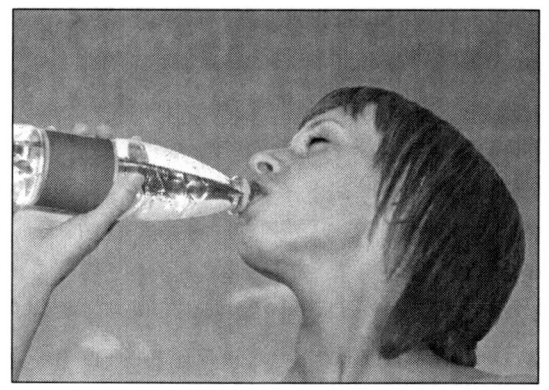

For this exercise, lie on your back on your mat or towel. Bend your knees and place your feet flat on the floor. Tighten your abdominal muscles and imagine that you are pulling your belly button through your back and into the floor. Place your arms either at your side or across your chest. Or, if your neck needs support, place your fingertips (not whole hands) *lightly* behind your head. Slowly contract your abdominal muscles and lift your shoulders off the floor, raising your chest to the ceiling. Your head, neck, and chest should be in alignment, and you should never tuck your chin or head into your chest. Imagine an apple between your chin and your chest, maintaining a steady distance. Slowly exhale as you lift and then slowly inhale as you lower. Remember, your hands should not pull your head in. Use your fingertips only for support, and focus on using your abdominal muscles to perform the movement.

If you are a beginner do two "sets" of 8 to 12 repetitions; raising and lowering together count as one repetition. As you become more advanced, slowly increase this to three sets of 12 to 15 repetitions. There is never a need to do more than 20 repetitions in a single set as this does not provide an increased benefit.

Again, remember to consult with your healthcare professional before beginning this exercise program. But once you are ready to begin, commit to performing these exercises three days a week with at least one day of rest in between each "workout" day to allow your muscles time to relax and recover. By doing these simple core exercises, you will be well on your way to developing a strong, healthy back!

Exercise Essentials: You CAN Achieve a Healthy Lifestyle

Experts agree on the importance of exercise to overall good health. And despite skyrocketing statistics on obesity and weight-related illnesses, the general public agrees on the importance of exercise as well. But as with any positive habit, there is a marked difference between a head-knowledge-assent to its importance and a determined commitment to make it a reality in one's own life.

This seems to be particularly true in the area of exercise. Each year, countless people place "start exercising" or "lose weight" at the top of their New Year's resolution list. And for a while, they stick to their commitment. It's a fact that health club regulars are well acquainted with the January rush of new members that comes in and takes over the gym equipment. The regulars are patient, however, as they realize that the majority of these newcomers will be strangers once again by March.

It's an unfortunate cycle that is repeated all too often. Yet, past failure does not have to equal future reality. And even if you are one of the many who have tried and failed before, you can make the decision *today* to begin a new healthy lifestyle by incorporating physical exercise into your daily routine. To provide you with the highest possible likelihood of success, here are five tips designed to get — and keep — you on the track toward good health.

Make Exercise A Regular Part of Your Calendar

Some of the busiest executives and public officials are regular exercisers. Like you, these men and women only have 24 hours per day, 168 hours per week, to work with. Yet somehow they manage to fit in all the responsibilities of their jobs and *still* make time to exercise. How do they do it? Ask any one of them, and you might be surprised at how many say that they literally schedule time in their calendars to exercise. These regular exercisers make an appointment with themselves, and then they let nothing get in the way of that appointment.

Whether you are a busy executive running a corporation or a work-at-home mom raising the next generation, your schedule is undoubtedly busy. Make the decision to schedule regular time into your day to take care of YOU. Many mothers will actually hire a babysitter in order to be able to exercise. And they reap the rewards many times over in good health, increased energy, and greater emotional wellbeing. So whatever your occupation, make exercise a regular part of your calendar.

Dress the Part

Many beginning exercisers dread the thought of going to a gym or fitness club because they imagine that everyone will be in tight spandex with bulging muscles. Unfortunately, this image, only sometimes true in reality, sends the message that you have to dress a certain way to exercise. In reality, however, the best clothing for fitness workouts is clothing that is comfortable and loose-fitting. It should allow you to move freely while not draping so much that it gets in the way of movement.

Watch Your Foundation

The surface on which you exercise is very important as it provides the foundational support for your movements. Select a firm surface that is solid yet comfortable. For back exercises, a carpeted living room floor will suffice; if the carpet is thin, try placing a mat or a towel on the floor for added support. Never perform back or other exercises on a soft surface such as a bed or couch, as these will not provide the support or stability your body needs.

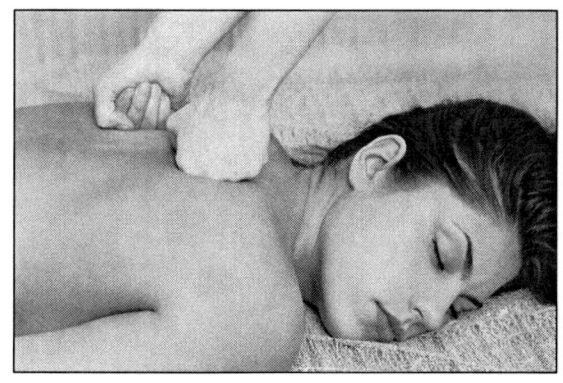

Quality over Quantity

All of us have that natural desire to go farther, to do more, to perform better. But in exercise (as in many things), quality is more important than quantity. When you are performing an exercise, it is better to practice proper form and perform the movement in a slow and controlled manner than race to get as many repetitions completed as possible without regard to form. Not only will the latter prove to be ineffective, it can also actually result in injury. So pay close attention to the form and movement of each exercise. Make sure you perform each repetition smoothly with no sudden or jerking motions. And if you find that by doing the exercise properly you are only able to complete 6 repetitions as opposed to 8, 10, or 12, that's ok! Exercise is a process, and while today you may only be able to do 6, with time you'll find your strength increasing if you commit to doing the exercises properly.

Progress at Your Own Pace

Perhaps our greatest enemy in exercise progression is the self-imposed "need" to be "better" than someone else. If we're not careful, this may cause us to try to progress faster than our bodies are able. For example, jumping suddenly from one set of 6 repetitions to three sets of 12 repetitions can place too much strain on your developing muscles and actually may result in an injury that keeps you sidelined for days or weeks. Remember, you are not in a competition. Listen to your body, and progress slowly at your own pace. You may find, too, that one week you progress and then the next week you are back to where you were two weeks prior. And this is ok, too. Keep the big picture in mind, and remember that fluctuations are normal. In the end, your goal is not a certain number of sets or repetitions but a healthy back.

If you commit to putting these five simple steps into practice, it will not be long before you begin to reap the rewards of the wonderful health benefits that a regular exercise program provides.

EXERCISES

1. Lower Back Stretch #1: Seated Flexion (forward bending)

Starting Position

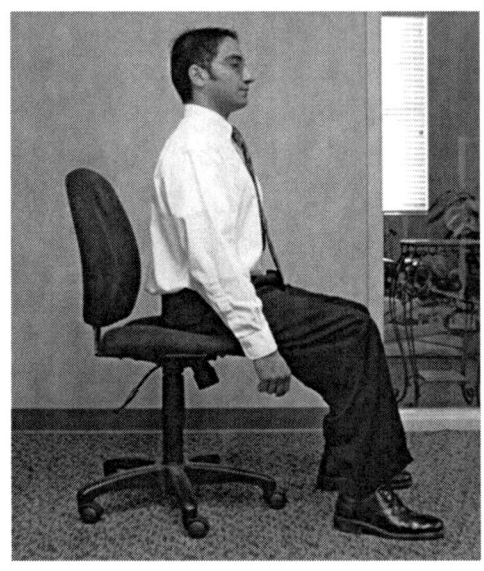

Stretching Position

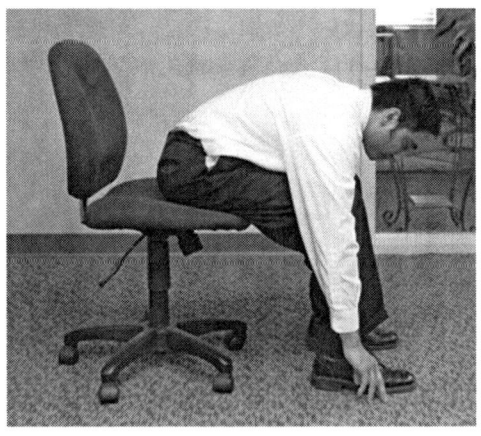

Start in a seated position. Slowly bend forward. You will start to feel a slight stretch in your lower back. Make sure you breath and go as far as comfortable. Hold for 30 seconds. And repeat four times, once a day.

2. Lower Abdomen Exercise #1: Draw – In

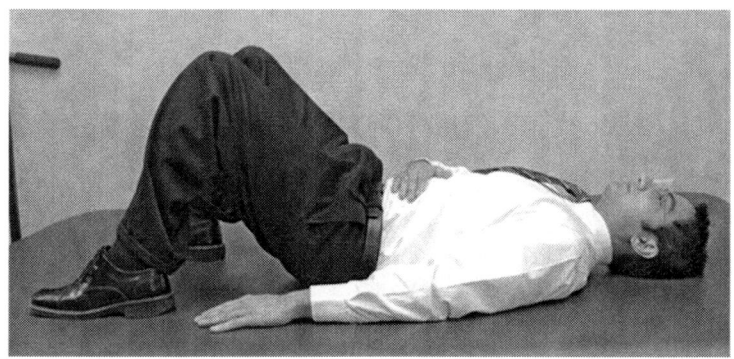

Start in a lying position. Slowly pouch your stomach out while you breath in. Then slowly exhale and draw your abdomen inwards towards your spine. Pretend you are trying to have your navel touch your spine. Make sure you keep breathing while holding that position for 10 seconds, repeat 4 times. You can do this exercise through out the day, but at least 4 times.

3. Lower Abdomen Exercise #2: Reverse Crunch

Starting Position

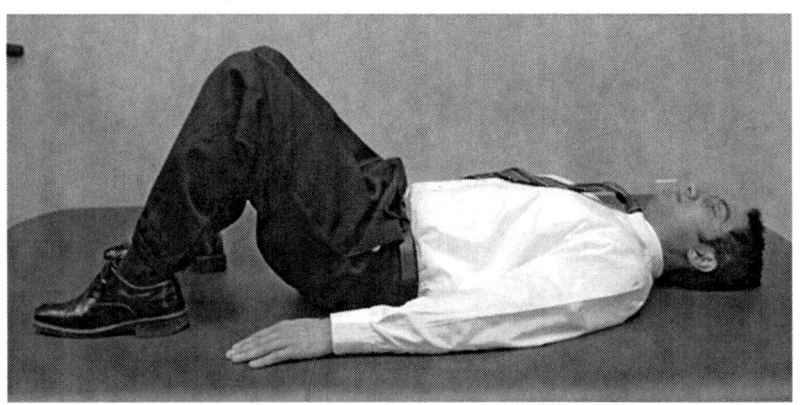

Final Position

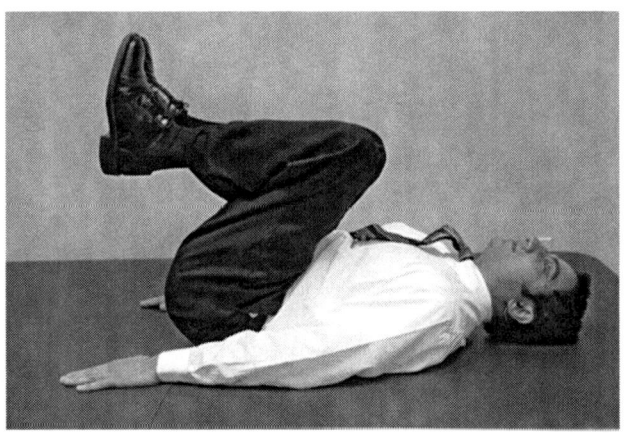

Start in a lying position on the floor with knees bent and arms at your side for support. Start contracting the muscles of your lower abdomen and slowly bring your knees towards your chest. It is important to contract your lower abdomen muscles and not just push off with your arms. Hold at the top position for 10 seconds and squeeze those lower abdomen muscles to really activate them. Then slowly lower your legs to starting position. Repeat 4 the motion times, 4 times per day.

4. Hip Flexor (Illopsoas) Stretch #1: Standing Hip Flexor

Starting Position   Stretching Position

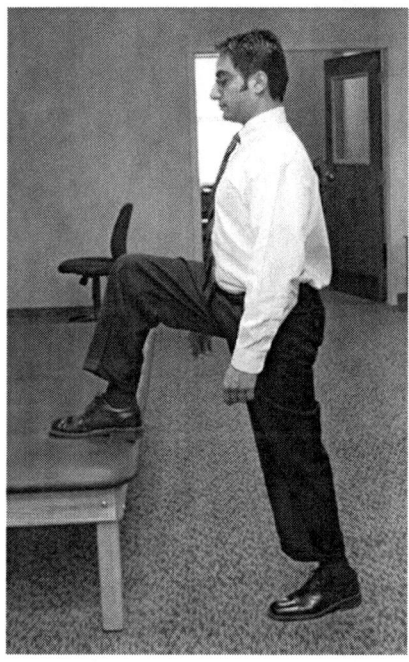 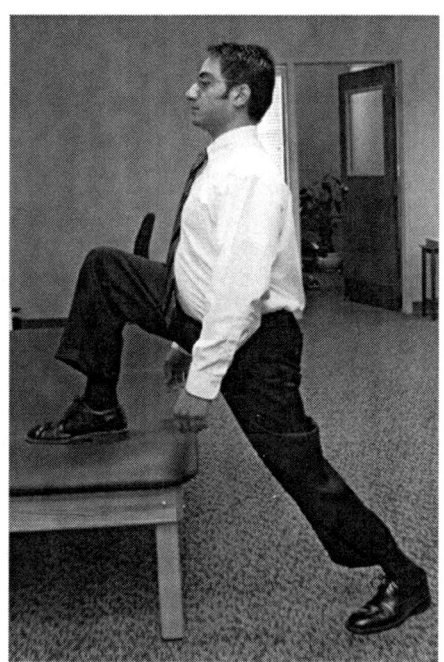

Start in a standing position. Have one leg on an elevated surface like a stair step and the other leg straight. Lean forward as if you were doing a lunge exercise. You will start to feel a nice stretch in the hip flexors. Go to a comfortable point and hold for 30 seconds. Repeat 4 times. Perform at least once per day.

5. Hip Flexor (Illopsoas) Stretch #2: Standing Hip Flexor #2

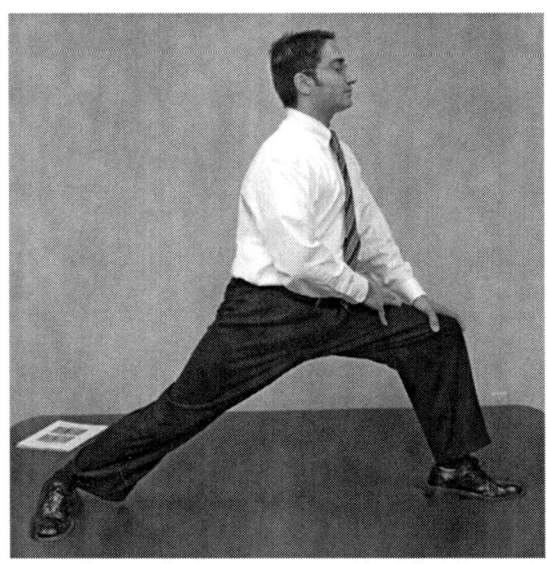

Start in a standing position. Lunge forward bending the front leg and keeping the back leg straight. Make sure not to have your knee pass your toe. That will put extra pressure in your knee. You can also hold on to something stable (like a wall, or chair) to help with balance. Hold for 30 seconds and stretch the other side. Do this 4 times for each hip flexor.

6. Bridge-Exercise: Pelvic Lift

Starting Position

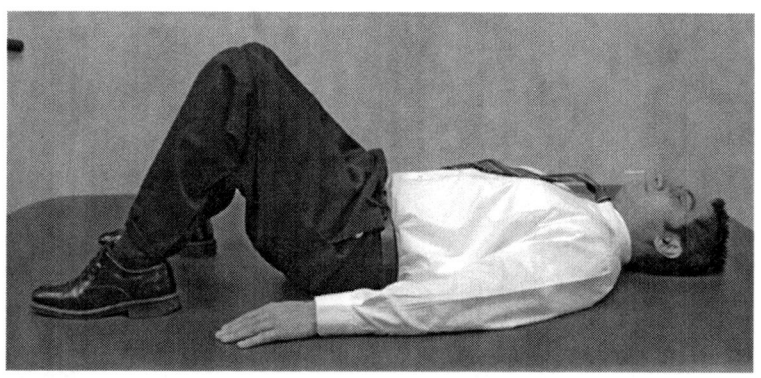

Bridge Position

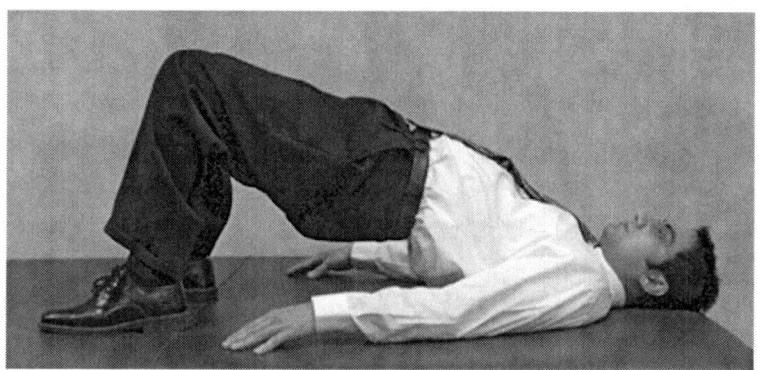

Start by lying on your back with both knees bent. Have your feet flat on the floor at about shoulder width apart and arms at your side. Slowly raise your hips bit by bit. Try to raise your hips without arching your back. Once you get to a comfortable position hold for 5 second and squeeze your gluts. Slowly lower your hips to the starting position. Repeat 10 times, performing it at least once per day.

7. Quadriceps Stretch

Starting Position

Stretching Position

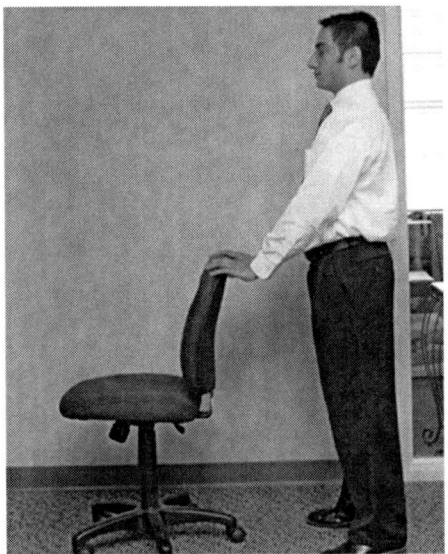 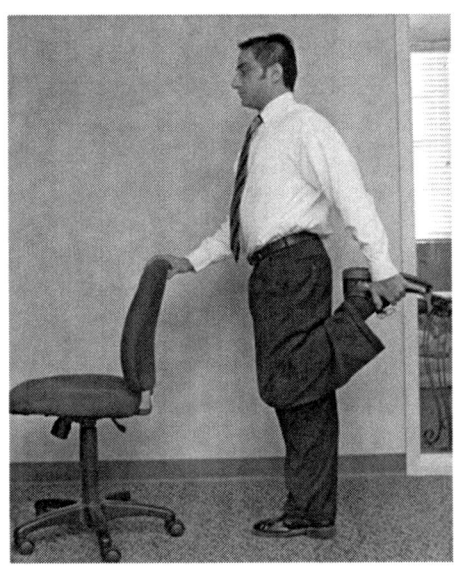

Start at a standing position holding to anything for balance. Feet should be shoulder width apart with toes forward. Slowly flex your lower leg and reach back and grab your foot. Gently pull your feet towards your gluts and hold for 30 seconds. Repeat 4 times at least once per day.

8. Inner Thigh Stretch

Starting Position

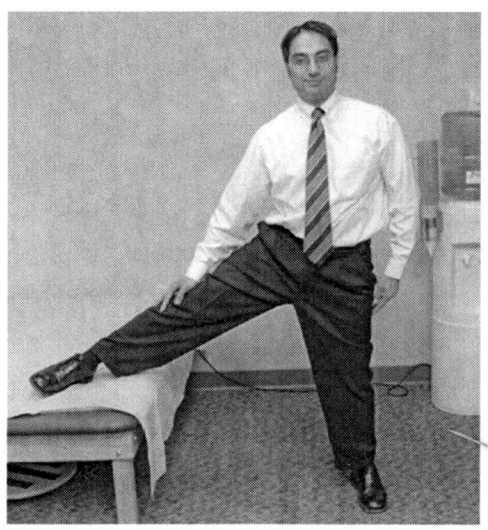

Stretching Position

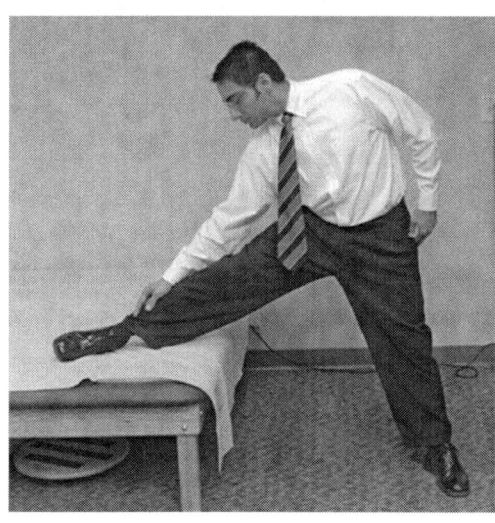

Begin in a standing position. Place the leg that you want to stretch on a elevated position like a chair or stair steps. Slowly lean toward the side of the elevated leg. Hold for 30 seconds and repeat 4 times.

9. Side Stretch

| Starting Position | Final Position |

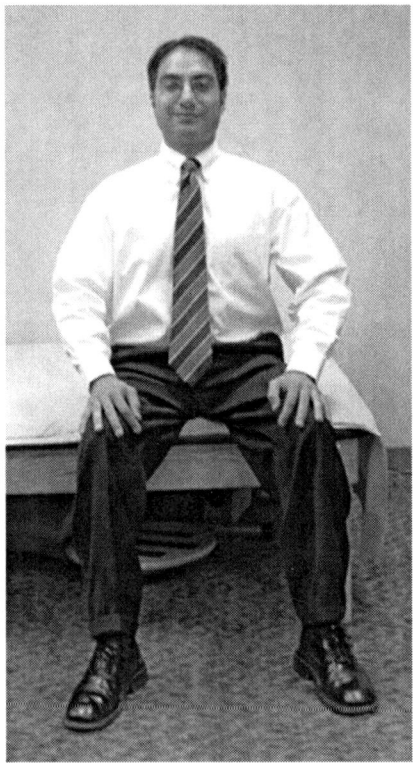 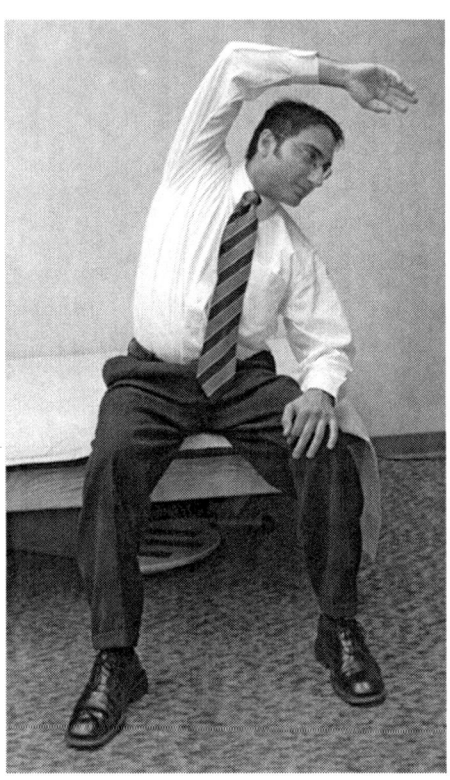

Begin in a seated position. Stretch one arm over your head and bend your upper body to the opposite side. Do not twist your body as you bend. Hold the stretch for a count of 10. Return to the starting position with your hands and arms at your side. Repeat 5 times and switch to the other side.

10. Hip Stretch #1

Starting Position

Second Position

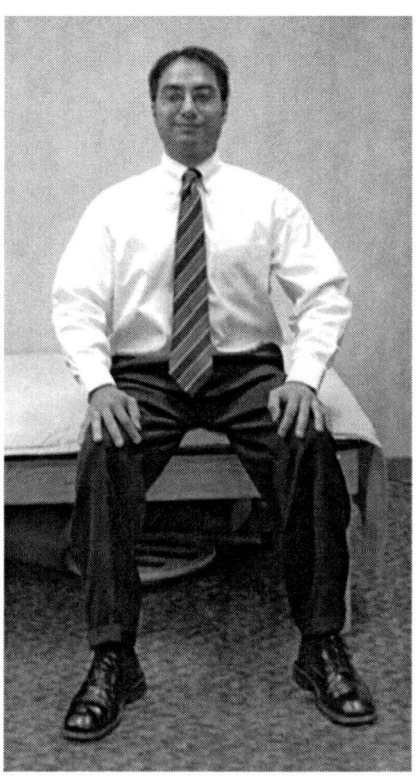
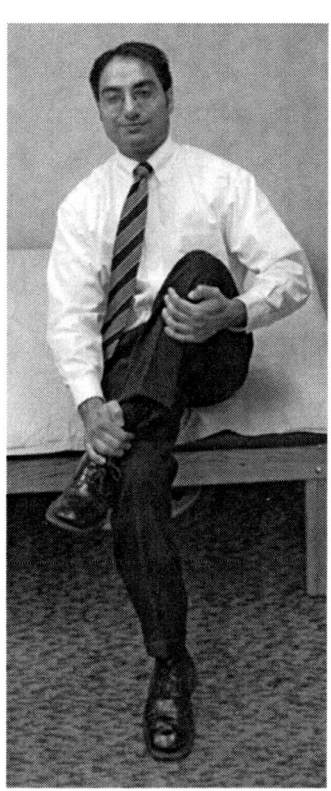

continues on next page

Final Position

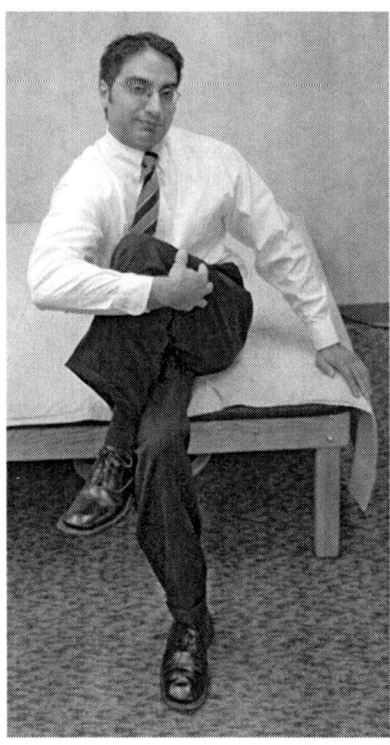

Begin in a seated position. Slowly bring the hip you want to stretch over and across your thigh. Then hold the bend leg at both the ankle and the knee at a comfortable position. Then slowly pull the bent leg inward toward your chest and then across your body. Slowly get back to the starting position and repeat. Hold for 10 seconds, repeat 5 time on both side.

11.   Hip Stretch #2

Starting Position

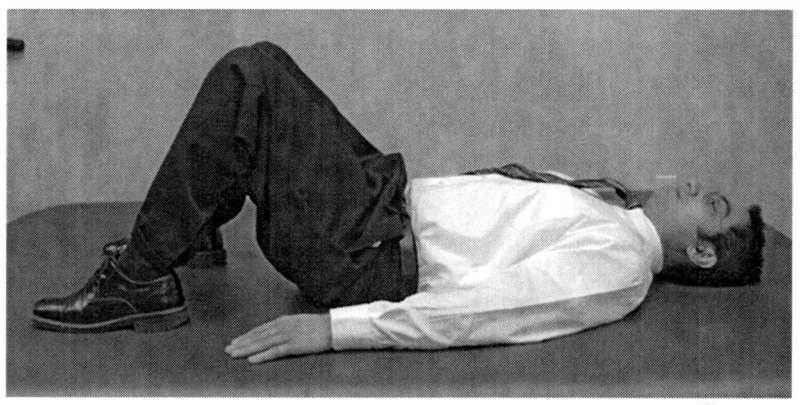

Stretching Position

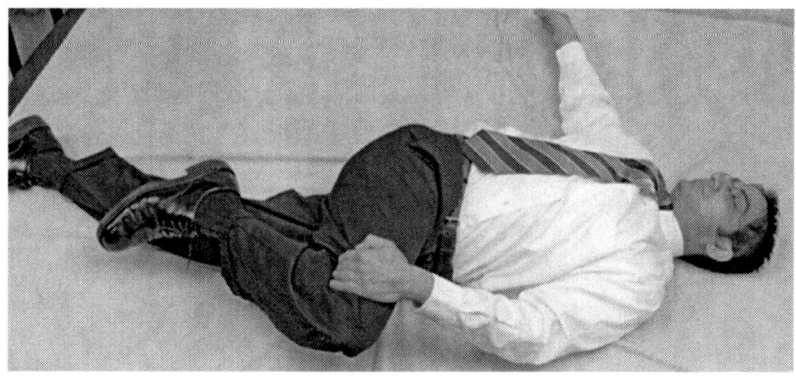

Start in a lying position on your back, knees together, feet on the floor. Take the hip you want to stretch and bring it over the other hip. Take the opposite hand and apply some downward pressure until you feel a good stretch. Hold for 30 seconds and return to starting position. Perform the stretch on the other side. Repeat 4 time on each side.

12. Glute Stretch

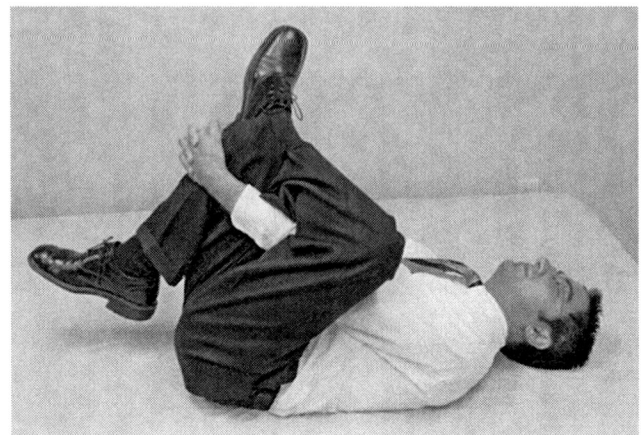

Begin by lying on your back with your knees bent. Cross one leg over the other at the knee and slowly bring the foot that is still on the floor up towards your chest. Grab your knee from under your leg that is crossed with both hands. Slowly release and uncross your leg and bring legs into starting position. Repeat the stretch using your other leg. Hold for 30 seconds and repeat 4 time on both sides.

13. Hamstring Stretch

Starting Position	Stretching Position
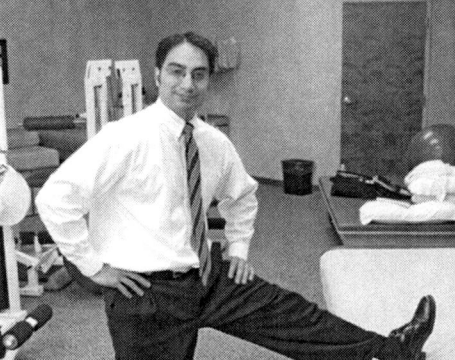	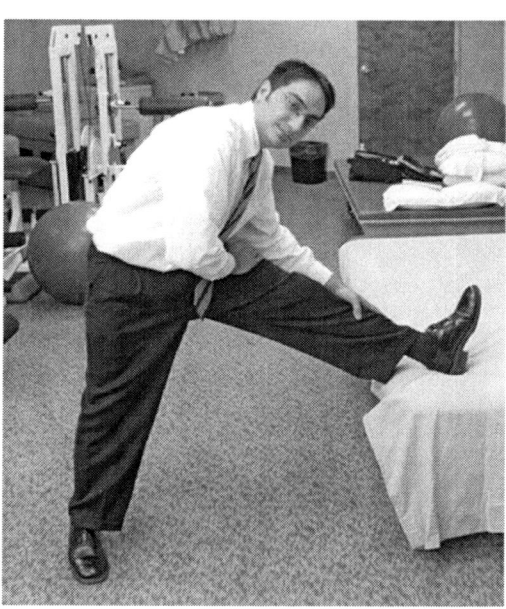

Start in a standing position with one foot on a chair or step. Hold something like a wall for support for better balance. Slowly reach for the toes. Get to a point where there a is a nice gentle stretch and hold for 30 seconds. Slowly come back to starting position and repeat on the stretch on the other leg. Perform 4 times

14. Abdomen Stretch

Starting Position

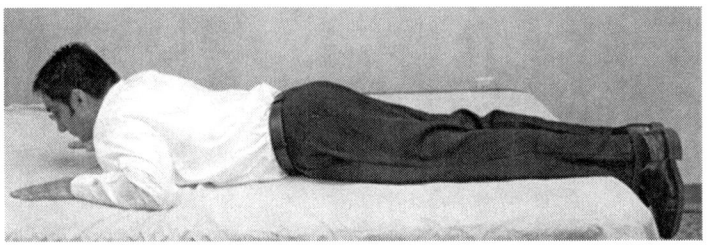

Second Position

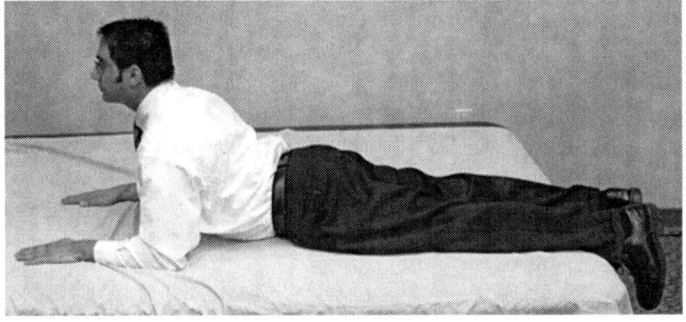

Final Position

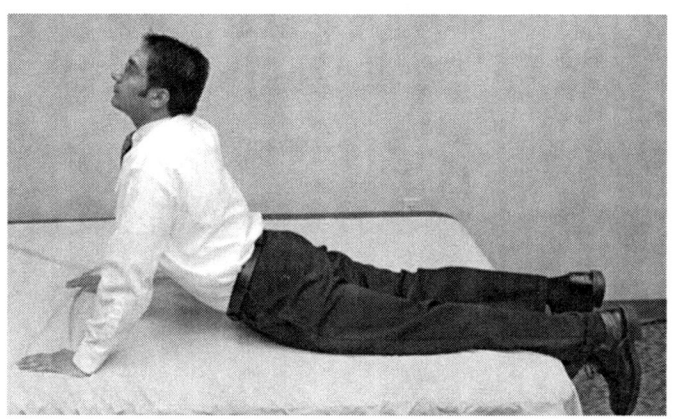

Start by lying on flat on your stomach with your feet slightly apart. Place your face near the floor and your hands palm down at face level. Use your arms to slowly push the top of your body to a resting position on your elbows. You may feel a tightness in your lower back or elbow. Hold this position for about 20 seconds. Then push up with your arms (still having your hands on the floor) as high as possible while keeping your hips and legs on the floor. Keep your back relaxed and hold the final position for 30 seconds. Slowly lower yourself back to the floor. Repeat 4 times.

For other books and programs by
Dr. Raj Banerjee, including

*"Dr. Banerjee's Guide to Hormone Imbalance:
Discover Simple Steps to Rebuild Your Life."*

FREE Video Newsletter, please visit:

http://www.DrBanerjee.com

You will also discover secrets:

- How to Reverse Chronic Fatigue

- How to Stop Depression Dead In It's Tracks

- How to Destroy Pain & Live Happy Without Pills

- How to Stop Dieting and Lose Weight Automatically

- Medical Secrets Doctors Never Mention

- *And Much, Much, More ...*

Please visit:
http://www.DrBanerjee.com

About the Author

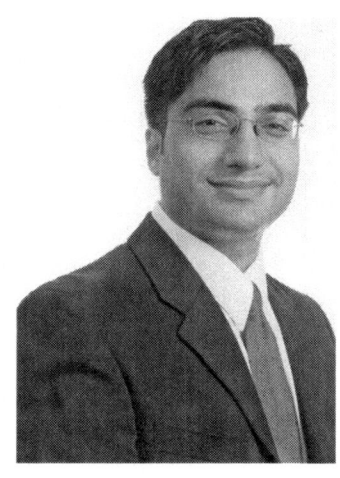

Dr. Raj Banerjee specializes in designing natural treatment programs for a wide range of health issues. Since 2000 he has successfully applied clinical nutrition protocols based on lab assessments for patients with hormone imbalances, food cravings, fatigue, depression, digestive distress and many other health complaints.

Dr. Banerjee maintains an active phone consultation practice designing nutritional programs and providing counseling to improve patients' health through diet and lifestyle modifications.

Dr. Raj Banerjee is a leading expert on health and wellness. In addition to practicing, he writes and speaks regularly to help business people make positive changes in their life. His entertaining presentations are filled with exciting and easy to use strategies. Help others to maximize their energy and minimize stress. Dr. Banerjee is available to speak to different groups and organizations.

For more information go to **www.drbanerjee.com**

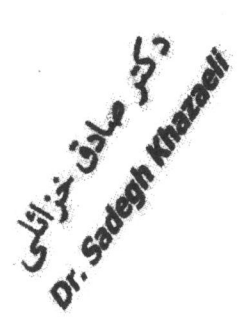

LaVergne, TN USA
15 September 2009
157914LV00001B/1/P